She Never Said Goodbye

George Vernon Ellison

What Readers are Saying

"Your story about Sara's problem, and your struggle to cope with the results, is a worthwhile story to tell. It is, of course, a disturbing situation and I sympathize with your situation. I have had a somewhat similar experience.

Unfortunately, until now, the vast majority of caregivers have no idea what is happening to their loved ones and the medical people are reluctant to utter the dreaded word 'Alzheimer's' until it has gone far enough to completely confuse and frustrate the ones observing. Now they will have some warning."

Herb Baker, retired engineer

"Wow! What a love story! I was moved by the amount of love, admiration and dedication Vern has for Sara. Vern's continued support and physical presence in Sara's life is inspiring."

W. Ruiz, editor

"I'm mired in the emotions of this one. Mercy. It touches on many levels for me. My Grandmother had this disease and my mother suffered enormously taking care of her for several years. A very, very painful disease for all involved. I'm so glad I'm reading this book, it is helping me understand my grandmother and have more compassion for what my mother went through. I only wish my mother could have read this book."

Pam Thomas, painting contractor

"Your book will be so helpful for many caregivers. As I read it, I immediately thought of my sister in law, who is a Alzheimer's caregiver and could use this kind of information.

Roger Granbo, retired executive

I think She Never Said Goodbye *is mandatory reading for anyone in what might look like a long-term caregiver situation...."*

M. Taglierii, artist and former publishing executive

She Never Said Goodbye

... My wife's disappearance
down a road of no return - Alzheimer's

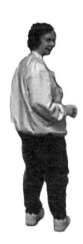

George Vernon Ellison
Loy Young

Aquarius House Press
Vista, California

Aquarius House Press
PO Box 1241
Vista, California 92085
760-758-7004 Fax: 760-758-8283
Email: AquariusHouse@aol.com
website: www.AquariusHousePress.com

Author - George Vernon Ellison
Co-Author and Writing Coach - Loy Young
Cover Design and Illustrator - Francine Dufour
Editor - Wendy Ruiz

Printed in the United States of America
First Printing February 2000

10 9 8 7 6 5 4 3 2 1
Library of Congress Catalog Card Number 00-190041
ISBN: 1-882888-51-0 - Hardback
ISBN: 1-882888-52-9 - Paperback

She Never Said Goodbye is dedicated to my beloved Sara, whose constant smile warms my heart and to our grandsons, Ethan Sheldon and Kyle Tristan Prager.

ACKNOWLEDGMENTS

As with most meaningful and heartfelt projects, many people gave of their time, wisdom and expertise to help us.

First we would like to thank the reviewers, we chose people we believed would be like you, the reader, to review our book. They are people who have good friends or family members that have gone through, or are going through, similar situations. The readers were quite helpful with their questions, comments, and suggestions. They are: Ray Stephens, Violet and Herb Baker, Roger Granbo, Bnai, Kathryn Hall, Mary Taglieri, Francine Dufour, Pam Thomas and Cody Buell.

Family members that were interviewed and provided priceless information and insight are:

Son - Corbin Ellison
Daughters - Amy Ellison Prager and Darby Ellison
Brother - Don Ellison
Sister in law - Pat Ellison
Sister - Virginia Ellison Weir
Sara's Mother - Shirley Gianelli
Sara's cousin - Daniel Raffetto

I'd especially like to thank the husbands and wives I talked to who were willing to share their own experiences with a spouse who had to be put into a home:

Mimi Lansberg
David Horowitz
Harold Mueller

Former journalist, Sam Marler, whose wife's father and mother have suffered from Alzheimer's, wrote stories about Sara and Vern of happier times, for us, thank you.

Thanks to author Bev Kruger in South Africa, Darby Ellison and Kathryn Hall who edited some of the Ellison's memoirs from which this book, *She Never Said Goodbye,* is taken.

And a special thanks to Wendy Ruiz for editing *She Never Said Goodbye.*

Thanks to Long-Term Health Insurance Specialist, Paul Riddle.

Special thanks to Sean Colin Ruiz who designed the *She Never Said Goodbye* Internet website to provide caregivers with a source of information regarding Alzheimer's disease, as well as providing a place to let others know about this important book. Please see us at http://www.AquariusHousePress.com

FOREWORD

Today the scope of the Alzheimer's/dementia problem is estimated by the National Alzheimer's Association to be over 4.5 million Americans. The special need of Alzheimer's/dementia individuals will severely test the moral fabric of our society.

I wish to acknowledge the family caregivers of long-term care individuals suffering through the five to twenty year passage of Alzheimer's disease, they are the brave people who have the courage to make a difference and are truly the second victims of Alzheimer's disease. They must learn to cope with "a stranger in the house," and in some cases a hostile and combative loved one. For those involved, the road is long and painful as they bear witness to the loss of the mind of a love one.

Just as business requires organization and strategic planning, family caregivers of Alzheimer's disease individuals need a well planned Coping Program for their loved one and themselves.

She Never Said Goodbye is the bittersweet story of a man and a woman who meet, marry, raise three children and live the military life during the first part of their journey of life together.

It is a chronological diary of Sara's early onset of Alzheimer's disease, and of the frustrations that families experience without benefit of a diagnosis, and with physicians not using the words "Alzheimer's disease." It is shocking to learn that there is no treatment other than memory enhancement drugs or psychotropic medications for behavioral management.

The author has shared his life with Sara, the good and the difficult, and it represents the development of special care for special people. Individuals with dementia appear to be different from us, they have their own likes and dislikes, sense of humor and low moods, but most importantly, they do have a soul that needs nourishing. This book gently reminds us there is indeed a person, with a spirit to be nourished, hidden beneath the mask of dementia.

She Never Said Goodbye carries a compelling message that will assist others to cope with the emotional upheaval of Alzheimer's disease and to better understand the anxiety and needs of their loved one.

It is a story of true and honest love, and one brave man's strength in surviving the impact of Alzheimer's disease.

Joy Glenner
President/CEO
The George G. Glenner Alzheimer's Family Centers, Inc.
San Diego, California

Contents

Preface

She Never Said Goodbye is the story of Sara's, and my, struggle with Alzheimer's. Sara is my beloved wife of thirty-seven years. She seldom speaks now, and then, just two or three words, yet with her contribution of the letters and scrapbooks she kept of our lives throughout the years, it's almost as if my Sara is telling our story right along with me.

Years ago, when I realized something was terribly wrong, I began taking notes on 3x5 cards to document the strange events happening in our life together. The woman I was married to, who had raised our children with me, seemed to disappear.

She never said goodbye.

Throughout the day, Sara claps her hands in front of her or on her body. Sometimes I think she's playing "patty cake, patty cake," a favorite game she played with our children long ago.

Although Alzheimer's is a disease that's usually equated with the elderly, there are a few early-onset cases like Sara's. The elderly often come down with the disease so late in life that they rarely go through all the symptoms equated with Alzheimer's. They die of other age related maladies, therefore there aren't a lot of case studies available showing all the stages and symptoms that people with Alzheimer's progress through.

This documentation contains several years discovery of what Alzheimer's can mean to a family whose wife and mother slowly disappears into an abyss from which there is no return. Sara was only in her early fifties when she became confused, depressed, and started losing her memory. Today, as we begin this century, Sara is sixty-four.

I've purposely left in some of the maddening repetition of events and dialogs in the hope you might get the feeling for what the disease does to someone's mind and the affect it could have on you if you are trying to care for the one you love.

She Never Said Goodbye is about Alzheimer's, it is also the story of how my unconditional love for Sara did not end as her mind began to shut down. My love has continued, with an emphasis on our vows of "in sickness and in health." To continue the closeness that we have had throughout the years, I had to discover other aspects of Sara—her feelings and her spiritual presence. I continue to document Sara's life, writing my observations on the cards I carry in my shirt pocket.

My life has been one of service, with twenty years in the Marine Corps and another seventeen teaching in the California Community College system. I know Sara would also like to continue to help others, even in her condition. She spent most of her life, even while raising our children, helping others as a compulsive, compassionate, professional volunteer. She drove the elderly on shopping trips and to medical appointments, taught children to read, baby sat, and participated in endless school activities and volunteer organizations.

I hope that by sharing the experiences we went through, it may help other people avoid some of the mistakes we made due to being unprepared and uninformed. Even the word Alzheimer's wasn't used when we started our journey.

Today Alzheimer's disease is the fourth leading cause of death among adults after heart disease, cancer, and strokes. Unlike the other diseases that can be identified by simple diagnostic tests, Alzheimer's, particularly in its very early stages, often remains a mystery to those with it, and around it.

You read heartwarming stories of people who recover from strokes, live happy lives after heart surgery, or beat cancer. But when faced with the less fashionable killer, Alzheimer's, you have to sadly come to terms with the knowledge that right now there is no recovery, no turning back, and no hope. It's a disease that presently has no cure. Dealing with facts as harsh as these are emotionally devastating. How can one cope with something that has no solution?

The research on Alzheimer's is really just beginning. Just since I've been writing this book, new scientific discoveries have been made. Still, these early breakthroughs deal with only how to delay the onset of the disease or to help those with early symptoms. No cures as yet!

If your loved one is diagnosed, you will need to learn a whole new world of information. To do that, you could find yourself spending enormous sums on doctors, lawyers, counselors, educational seminars, and financial advisors. This is money you're going to need for your loved one's care—or your own.

Hopefully this book will be helpful as I've written about the challenges we went through: discovery, medical intervention and evaluation, research, legal considerations, financial ramifications, and the continual decision making I had to deal with in facing the declining health of my Sara. In writing this story, I've carefully changed most names and places to respect the privacy of those involved.

Alzheimer's is a long-term disease, sometimes dragging on for as long as twenty years before death releases the spirit. This book does not end our situation.

I must admit that I wrote this book to restore and maintain my own sanity, as well inform others of the struggle. As I reviewed our lives, I was able to remember the happier, more fulfilling times we shared together.

Vern Ellison

Part One
The Years Before

Chapter 1

She Came in Silence

*T*o begin this story we need to start with Sara's conception. She was conceived in love by parents who very much wanted her, which may account for her gentle, loving nature. Her mother perceived Sara's nine months in the womb as normal and it was a time of close bonding between mother and unborn child.

Her birth on December 9, 1935, at 8:45 p.m. was anything but normal. Anxiety, suspense, and worry marked her birth. Her spirit came in silence, never uttering a sound until long past midnight. Her breathing was faint. *Would Sara make it?* No one really knew. Sara's parents, Dick and Shirley Patterson, had incompatible blood types, her father was Rh positive and her mother was Rh negative. Many babies like Sara, often called blue babies, never made it beyond the delivery room.

Her spirit finally settled into her tiny body about 12:45 a.m. She let out a small, delicate, fragile sound, letting her parents know she would indeed live. Those attending her birth let out great sighs of relief.

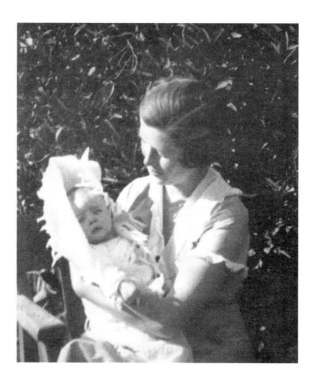

Shirley decided to name her daughter, Sara, without the "h." She wanted her daughter to be special and throughout her life Sara would say, "My name is Sara without the 'h'."

Sara Joyce Patterson was born in Placerville, California, located in the foothills of the Sierras east of Sacramento. This one-time mining town had its beginnings during the California gold rush and was originally known as Hangtown. Today a dummy hanging in front of a popular local bar commemorates Placerville's origins.

Settlers arrived in Hangtown during the gold rush with dreams of striking it rich. Sara's maternal grandparents arrived during that time, hoping to make their fortune. The real wealth in Hangtown, soon to become Placerville, turned out to be the families who came, stayed to raise children and grow the crops that Placerville's climate was ideal for growing, especially apples and pears.

Sara's father, Dick Patterson, was 5'10", with a great athletic build and a personable smile that won everyone over. Dick was an only child from Illinois. His father was a dentist in the Army so the

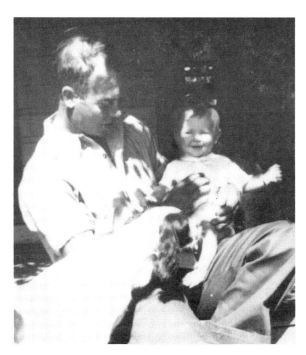

family moved around a great deal. When he arrived in Placerville, his parents lived in San Francisco and his father was assigned to The Presidio. His mother was a homemaker.

When Dick's mother was in her eighties, she would lose her memory and be put into a nursing home. In all probability she had Alzheimer's disease. People said she was senile or had "lost her mind."

At this time in our story though, Dick's mother was still vibrant and full of life. Dick had come to Placerville from the Bay area looking for a pear ranch. He stayed at the Raffles Hotel while he was looking for property. At the hotel he noticed a mural of a deer on the wall and greatly admired it. He remarked, "The painting of that deer is so lifelike. Who painted it?" When someone pointed out Shirley, the waitress and niece of the owner of the hotel, he asked to meet her.

Shirley, a petite and most attractive blond, may have been working as a waitress, but in her heart dwelled an artist. She painted whenever and wherever she could.

Dick admired a lot more about Shirley than just her painting. It wasn't long before he asked Shirley to marry him. He was ten years older than she and anxious to begin a family. She agreed, and after they married moved to his newfound pear ranch on the outskirts of Placerville.

After Sara's birth, her parents decided to gamble with fate one more time. They really wanted a baby brother for Sara. They were not so lucky this time. They did have a baby boy, but like Sara, he did not let out a sound for four grueling hours and then, the only sound they heard was the baby gasping for his breath — which soon stopped. Shirley still gets tears in her eyes as she tells the story of burying their baby boy at the top of a hill on their pear ranch.

They tried once again knowing the odds were clearly not with them. This time Shirley never made it to the delivery room, but was rushed to the hospital, hemorrhaging badly. She nearly died and the baby girl in her womb never had the chance to draw a breath of air or make a sound.

That was the end of Shirley's dream of having more children with Dick, which truly saddened her. Shirley equated being a mother with her destiny in life. Sara, like her father, would be her father's only child.

Being the only child wasn't the only similarity between father and daughter. Sara had a smile that won hearts, just like her father.

When Sara was about a year old, her mother recounts that they almost lost her to a bout of pneumonia. Luckily, the same doctor who delivered her came out to the ranch and was able to save her. Throughout Sara's life she would remain susceptible to upper respiratory infections.

Sara's mother recalls that her daughter was adored through her childhood. It didn't matter whether it was family or a stranger. Once when they went to San Francisco to get Sara's picture taken, the store owner asked if he could put her picture in the window for all to see, she had a smile and a personality that drew everyone to her.

Sara was quite independent, she would run off by herself. One time in downtown San Francisco Sara took off by herself, scaring Shirley near to death.

To understand more of Sara's childhood and teen years, we can hear directly from Sara. Much later in her life, our youngest daughter, Amy, interviewed her to learn about her mother's childhood and early adult years.

The interview showed a keen insight to Sara's personality and the times she grew up in, I'm including some excerpts.

ORAL HISTORY PROJECT
by Amy Ellison, Lincoln Middle School, 1982

The subject of my interview was Sara Ellison, my mother.

AMY: Could you tell me what it was like living on a farm and what you did there?

SARA: Well it was a lot of fun living on a farm. I was rather lonely because I was an only child but I played with all the animals. We had lots of horses (I had my own horse), and pigs which I used to name. I played dolls with them and dressed them. I'd run my dad's tractor in the orchards and helped milk the cows. We also had chickens and peacocks. It was a big occasion when we had someone come and visit.

AMY: Where were some of the places you lived up until high school?

SARA: I lived in Placerville, California, until I was five. And then we lived in New York City for a year. From New York we moved back to Placerville and then we moved to Portland, Oregon, for a few years and that's where my parents were divorced. My mom and I and my adopted baby brother moved back to Placerville. Then after quite some time my mom remarried and we moved to Fort Worth, Texas. It wasn't long before I had a new baby brother.

AMY: Do you think moving around a lot affected you?

SARA: Well, I was lonesome, but I seemed to make new friends quickly so it didn't really bother me. I always missed my cousins in Placerville but I went to visit people every summer from the time I was ten. So, I really got to see everyone.

AMY: How did you spend your summers?

SARA: Each summer after I moved to Texas, I would fly out to my dad's house in Portland and I would fly all by myself in an airplane. The stewardesses took care of me. One of the times I got very, very frightened on the airplane. That was before jets. These were propeller airplanes and it took forever to fly from Fort Worth to Portland. So when it came time to come home at the end of August I wouldn't go. I had to travel by train. My dad got train fare for me. I had what they called a bedroom. And I went in this bedroom across country and my father bought me this darling little golden cocker puppy to keep me company. It took me four days and three nights going to Texas. It was fun except I was kind of frightened. I had all my meals served in my room. But it was fun riding on a train and it would kind of rock you to sleep.

AMY: What kind of fast food places were there?

SARA: When I was growing up there were no fast food places like there are now. You would go to a drive-in and if you were very lucky you got to have a root beer float or a sundae or a banana split. But there were none of the things we have now. Let's see. A root beer float cost 25 cents and it was a real treat when we got to have one of those. Pizza came out, or started to be popular, when I was a senior in high school. My mom had a graduation party for my girl-friends and she made pizza but it was not at all like it is now. It was very good, and it was exciting because I was the only one who had a pizza party.

AMY: What kinds of jobs were available for students?

SARA: The only thing that you could really do was baby sitting. Or you could work in the department stores over Christmas. There were no fast food places. Now one of the other things that I remember is that you could work as an usher in a movie. Those were available. But there were very few jobs. So in the summertime, after I graduated from high school, they always asked you, "Are you going back to school?" If you said, "Yes, I'm going back to school in the fall," you never got a job. But if you didn't tell the truth maybe you could get a job. My dad was very nice to me and he let me work for him. I worked in the advertising section of the Oregon-Washington-California Pear Bureau. I mailed out advertisements and things like that so if it hadn't been for him, I probably wouldn't have had a job during the summer.

AMY: Tell me about some of the fads and fashions that were around when you were a teenager.

SARA: Well we wore saddle shoes, Angora sweaters, and had our socks rolled down. In California the boys wore trousers called "grays" and the girls wore plaid skirts and long-sleeved shirts. That was in California, not in Texas. They dressed up a lot in Texas. Frilly clothes and so forth. In California it was more sport clothes. In Texas you always wore earrings and in California you never did.

AMY: What was your families socioeconomic standing?

SARA: Well, I would say that in the beginning when we were on the farm, we just made ends meet. Then my father started in managing the Pear Bureau, and we were fine. We were middle class. Then when my parents got divorced that was kind of hard again although my father took care of me quite nicely. When my mother remarried, she married a very frugal man. He was very nice and things were adequate. My father would spoil me and send me nice, nice things and he'd come through town and take me out to dinner and buy me any clothes I wanted. He even gave me a fur coat when I graduated from high school. I absolutely couldn't believe it was me, so I was a spoiled child.

AMY: Tell me about your feelings toward the bombing of Pearl Harbor.

SARA: The bombing of Pearl Harbor took place when I was five and a half years old and I remember it vividly. We were ice skating in Central Park and we had just gone in to have hot chocolate when we heard it on the news. My parents became very upset. I was really too little to know

what was happening but I caught their feelings. Shortly af-
ter that we had air raid practices and those were very fright-
ening back in New York. When we were in school, big air
raid sirens would sound and we would have to file out from
our private school and go between the tall buildings. Dur-
ing the day we had air raid drills and at night we had black-
outs. You would have to draw your curtains and get under
the tables and that was scary.

AMY: What precautions were taken and what were
some of the effects?

SARA: For air raids the big street lights were painted
over in dark colors. We turned them off at night so planes
flying over couldn't spy on the cities. We had maps of where
to go to air raid shelters and bombing drills. A lot of our
food supply was short and I can remember standing in line
for bread. We had absolutely no bubble gum, but I was lucky
because my cousins owned a variety store. When they did get
a shipment of bubble gum, my cousins and I got the first
share. The other thing there was absolutely no butter. What
we got was Nucco. It was white, with the consistency of but-
ter. And then there was this little pellet that you were to
squish into the margarine. It was supposed to color the mar-
garine to make it look like butter. It was ghastly! We went
without plenty of foods during the war. And there was gas
rationing and you couldn't buy new tires. You didn't go on
trips. If you needed a new tire, you had to settle for retreads.
Everyone was very patriotic and saved aluminum and ev-
erything for the war effort. I'm sure there were other things,
but I was too young to remember. We had ration books, but
I don't remember what was rationed except for gas.

****

Amy included these observations after the interview:

The Korean War happened when Sara lived in Texas,
next to Carlswell Air Force Base. Jets flew over her house

and everything shook. She waved to the pilots because they were so low.

Families with phones usually had party lines. Out on the ranch, Sara had a phone on the wall where you would crank the handle and tell the operator a number such as 228J. In college you just had to pick it up (the receiver) and tell the operator you needed a certain number.

Televisions came on sale when she was in the seventh grade. Her family did not own a TV, but the family next door did. When she went over there to baby sit she watched TV all day. There were only two channels and the only program she recalled was Howdy Doody.

Most rich people in Forth Worth had telephones, maids, and butlers. Not everyone enjoyed such luxuries. Most rich people owned a Cadillac.

Drugs and smoking were not a problem when Sara was growing up. Drugs weren't freely available. Few people smoked cigarettes and they were not the types you associated with. If you did, you were tarred with the same brush.

The average school had the same subjects as now like typing, sewing, and math. Now many alternatives exist, but way back then there were no special classes.

Asked for her impressions after interviewing her mother, Amy said, "Personally and emotionally I learned how hard it was for my mother to leave her father when her parents were divorced. She loved her father very much. People back then didn't get divorced often."

In an interview for this book, our eldest daughter Darby shared Amy's sentiments about Sara's childhood and its impact on her later life. Darby remembered that her mother often talked about her parent's divorce as the most devastating, traumatic event of her childhood. Sara even blamed herself, thinking the divorce was her fault.

Sara adored her father and she never understood being separated from him for any reason. She never really forgave her mother for divorcing her father, thus putting a strain on their relationship throughout their lives.

In later years, Sara would instill in our children the belief that they should never divorce, no matter what happened. She said, "When you marry, you stay married." As an adult, Darby witnessed Sara hiding in a closet crying because a close friend was getting a divorce.

Darby recounted another trauma in Sara's childhood that was closely linked to the divorce. Shirley moved back to Placerville with Sara and her adopted son, Dicky. Divorce carried a stigma directed more at the woman for a failed marriage.

Shirley decided to distance herself from the stigma by not working in Placerville, but in a nearby town. Instead of taking Sara and Dicky with her, she left them in the care of her mother in Placerville.

Sara was devastated by this perceived desertion by her mother. Decades later during arguments with her mother, the emotions usually went back to this time period. Sara would say accusingly to her Mother, "Don't you remember leaving me when I was small?"

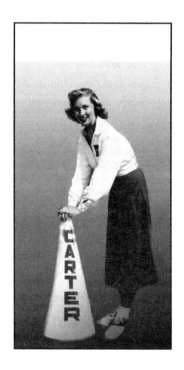

During high school in Fort Worth, Sara was quite active. She was a cheerleader for three years and served one year as the secretary of the Cheerleader's Club. She participated in the Dance Club, Junior Red Cross, and the Girl's Tennis Team. She was always an extremely popular member of her class.

Her senior yearbook is full of comments from friends and teachers about how friendly, nice, gracious, sweet, and cute Sara was. Everyone commented about her infectious smile.

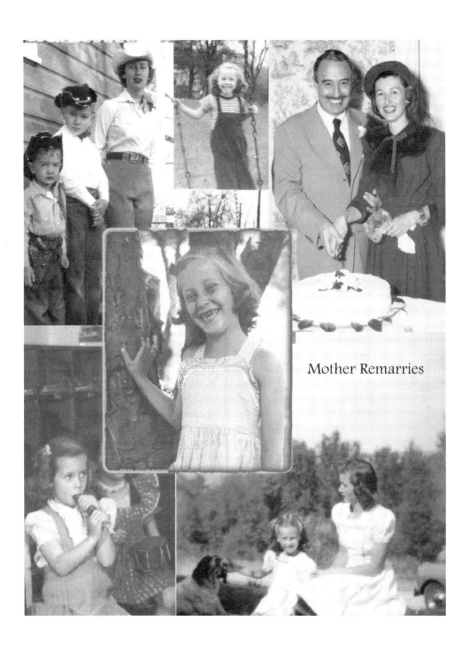

Mother Remarries

Chapter 2

Her Constant Smile
Captivates Me

O ne year older than Sara, I was born in Eugene, Oregon two days after Christmas on December 27, 1934, at 10:14 p.m. Named after my mother Georgia and my great grandfather, George Amy Stanton, I became George Vernon Ellison.

Our President was Franklin D. Roosevelt. The entire U.S. population was 126,485,000. St. Louis won the World Series over Detroit and Cavalcade was the winner of the Kentucky Derby. The most outstanding movie was *It Happened One Night*. The best actor and actress respectively,

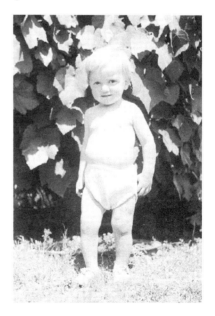

were Clark Gable and Claudette Colbert. The Kraft Music Hall Radio Show won awards that year and the favorite book was *Goodbye Mr. Chips*.

Dust bowl storms hit the United States and many parts of the country suffered from the terrible drought. The Great Depression became worse than it already was.

By today's standards I would say prices were quite reasonable. A three bedroom house was $2,925, a new Ford car cost $535, and a gallon of gas was just nineteen cents. A one pound loaf of bread cost eight cents and a gallon of milk was forty-four cents. To keep things in perspective, the average income was just $1,237 a year.

My father was Chester Prentice Ellison, although he was called by one of several nicknames — Bud, Chet, or Slim. Dad was indeed slim, and at 6'1", attractive in a rugged Gary Cooper kind of way with deep set blue eyes offset by dark brown hair.

Like all kids in the Ellison family, Dad began his working career early. Out of the twelve children born, eight survived. One was stillborn, one lived only eleven days, one died at thirteen, and another at eighteen. Dad was fourth in the lineup of twelve. Surviving and eking out a living was what mattered. He had only a grade school education and remained a laborer throughout his life.

Dad struggled in his trade as a house painter. Whenever I see a homeless person with a sign saying "willing to work for food," I often think of my dad, as it was not uncommon for him to indeed do just that — work at anything for food to bring home to his family.

A smile from him was rare, but then he didn't think he had much to smile about, nor did he talk much. He was serious about life and worked hard to provide for us. He must have seen his job description in the family as fulltime provider.

My mother was one of six girls, a small family in comparison to my father's. Mother was number five, she was born Georgia Edith Pulley in Corvallis, Oregon, in 1912. Mom was medium height, 5'6", but next to dad, she always seemed small to me. Unlike my slim father, mother struggled with weight her entire life. I guess you could liken her looks to the popular actress, Shirley Booth.

Like Dad, she too rarely ever smiled, her approach to life was equally serious. When it came to talking though, she was just the opposite. No one ever got to stay a stranger with her—she'd ask every possible question until she knew everything about the former stranger.

As hard as dad worked at being a provider, mom matched his efforts in the home. Besides doing the cooking from scratch (with no jiffy mixes or microwave), she did the washing, ironing, cleaning and looked after us. How she found the time, I do not know, but she even managed to attend every school event we were involved in.

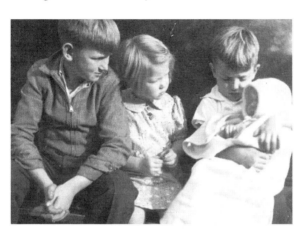

Our family was even smaller than my parents had been. There was my older brother, Donald, a younger sister, Virginia, my younger brother Paul, and myself. Mom lost a baby girl between my big brother and me.

An event that shaped my early life and probably influenced my whole response to the caregiver role I inherited with Sara, was the birth of my little brother Paul. Little Paul had beautiful blue eyes, the only one in the family to inherit Dad's deep set blue eyes. His story really pulled at our heartstrings.

In 1939 the Eugene Hospital had an iron clad policy that a baby could not be born in the hospital without a doctor present. Mother, responding to nature not hospital policies, began to give birth before the doctor arrived. The duty nurse dutifully halted the birth by pushing the little head back and kept it there until the doctor finally arrived. As a result, Paul suffered brain damage and would grow up with limited mental capacity. Malpractice suits weren't a way of life yet, so my parents didn't think of engaging a lawyer.

When little Paul was a youngster, we included him by putting him in a jumper and attaching the harness to a pole. Donald, my older brother, took one end of the pole and I'd take the other. Never able to utter a word, Paul had a constant smile on his face.

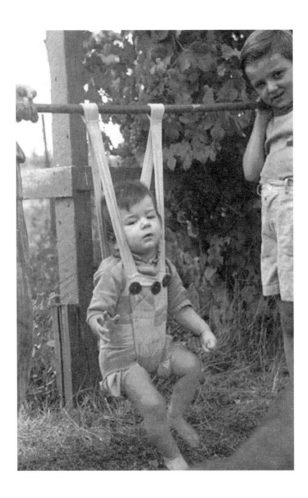

In 1943, when I was nine years old, we moved north some forty miles to Mom's Oregon birthplace, Corvallis. Even though it meant leaving behind all the Ellison aunts, uncles and cousins, I was happy to be moving to a place that seemed a lot better than what we had. 1601 Brook Lane was a mile from the Oregon State College campus. Our home was a small two bedroom house, with a large, enclosed porch and an attached woodshed, on nine acres. Even though the house was about the same as in Eugene, it felt so much bigger with the nine acres, instead of the previous half acre.

Our new homestead sat comfortably on the banks of the Mary's River and in the wintertime when it would freeze, Donald, Virginia and I would ice skate and have a great time.

As little Paul got older, it was increasingly difficult to take care of him. Although he could not open a door, he knew when one was not completely closed and he'd be off running like a shot. Boy, that little guy was fast!

All of us—my brother, sister and I—had a hard time catching him. There was no way our mother could ever catch him when he got away. Each time Paul escaped from our home and disappeared, we all panicked, Mom most of all. Out in the country where we lived there were so many places to hide. On occasion a kindly neighbor would see him running loose and bring him home to us.

On one escape Paul headed for the river with my brother Donald and me in hot pursuit. Our mother was so scared she began to cry. This caused my parents to make a painful decision, although one that was necessary for his own safety, Paul had to be put in a home where he couldn't run away. Even though I understood the reason, it was a devastating experience for me. I don't remember even getting to say goodbye to him. He just disappeared from my life.

After my graduation from Corvallis High School in 1953, I attended Oregon State. I earned a total of nine varsity letters in football, wrestling, and track and field in high school, and I decided to continue with athletics in college. I pledged the Sigma Phi Epsilon fraternity and majored in natural resources, which was academically challenging and truly interesting. I also entered the reserve officers training program (ROTC).

Sara and I met during my junior year and Sara's sophomore year. Sara had wanted to attend college at the University of California-Berkeley because her cousins were going there, however, her father would only pay for her education if she went to college in Oregon where he still managed the Oregon-Washington-California Pear Bureau. *Oh how Fate has a way of matching people up together for its own reason.*

Sara was not particularly happy about this decision. She never really liked Oregon, it was too rainy for her. It took her a good year before she settled into her surroundings at Oregon State College. Fortunately, her outgoing personality, friendliness, and good looks allowed her to make many friends.

She joined the Kappa Alpha Theta sorority. Kappa Alpha Theta girls were known for their intellect and for being high achievers. During rush, Sara was thought to be rather scandalous for wearing earrings—even though that had been the fashion where she came from in Texas. In the end, they accepted her into the sorority despite the earrings.

Sara majored in home economics. She was clear that her career goal was to be a wife and mother.

I was dating one of her Kappa Alpha Theta sorority sisters when we met on a double date. Sara's smile captivated me from the very beginning. We went to the coast in Sara's date's two seater car. My date and I were hunkered down behind the seats with no room to move, exhaust fumes rolling in, and unable to see outside. It was quite a time.

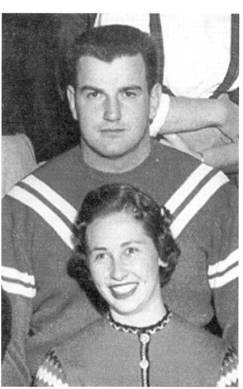

Shortly after that first meeting, I asked Sara out. She was a very attractive young woman with blonde hair, a smile forever on her face, very energetic, and always a pleasure to be with. I must admit, from the very beginning, there was a gentleness about her that made me want to take care of her. Over the next couple of years we dated off and on.

Then during the spring of my senior year, 1957, Sara and I became "pinned." That meant I gave her my fraternity pin to wear, which was often viewed as a sign of pre engagement. Sara and I were happy and really quite moved by the pinning.

I graduated in June of 1957 and was commissioned a second lieutenant in the U.S. Marine Corps. Although I had been a 12th round draft choice of the Pittsburgh Steelers of the National Football League, I was obligated for four years of service in the Marine Corps, due to my ROTC commitment.

After graduation, I headed for the East Coast, to attend the Marine Corps officer basic training in Quantico, Virginia. Sara found she didn't enjoy being pinned during her senior year of college. I was too far away to escort her to all the various activities so with no warning she gave my fraternity pin back along with a note telling me that I had a job to do in the Marines and I would be too far away for an unknown period of time. She even let me know that she didn't really like my career choice of the Marines. She never said goodbye, only a note. I admit, I felt disrespected and somewhat devastated.

The Marine Corps left me little time to lament—I was soon off to Lebanon, participating in an amphibious landing on July 15, 1958. Sara and I lost touch, but she stayed in my mind. I thought of her often.

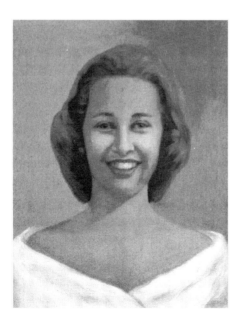

At one of our ports of call I ran across a portrait artist who would paint an oil painting from a photograph. His work looked quite professional. I opted to have him paint a portrait of Sara from a black and white photo I had. I wasn't really sure I'd ever see the final picture, but I decided to give it a chance. When I got back to the States, a package arrived. It was a beautiful colored oil painting of Sara. I must say I was impressed.

After college, Sara moved to San Francisco and became a bank teller. When I got transferred to Camp Pendleton, we got together a couple of times and had a really good time. I went up to San Francisco and we spent a day at the beach. I thought we were back on again, it was kind of like the old days. From all outward indications, we were both happy.

Shirley, Sara's mother, speaks of this time when Sara was living in San Francisco, as being quite fearful. Wolves were at her door trying to paw Sara constantly because of her good looks and personality. She put on quite a bit of weight, so much so, that in later years she would destroy all the pictures of that period showing her to be a little on the "chunky" side. Later, she would live a life of a woman of 110 pounds. A couple of pounds over, and she'd starve herself until it was resolved.

After a few weeks, Sara's mail began to dwindle, and it wasn't long before I got another note from her telling me she was getting married to her high school sweetheart and moving to Texas.

Excerpts dated February 13, 1961:

> *Dear Vern -*
>
> *It was nice to hear from you - after all the times you have called and I always seem to be up to no good. Vern, March the first I am getting married in Fort Worth, Texas. I am very happy Vern and such a fortunate girl. (Husband) and I went to high school together in Texas. All these years we have kept in touch off and on. He flew out for my birthday and asked Dad if we could marry. We had many wonderful times together and truly I wish to thank you. I hope we will keep in contact and I have the opportunity to introduce you to my husband. I want him to be your friend. Take care now and please keep a good head on your shoulders - The very best to you, Vern.*
>
> *Love, Sara*

Another goodbye from Sara. I must say I was surprised or even shocked to receive Sara's letter. I'd never heard Sara mention anything about her former high school sweetheart through all the years I'd known her. This time it looked final, my life was to continue without Sara. My heart felt heavy.

While Sara went off to Texas, I went to Adak, Alaska. *Where is that?* It is in the middle of the Aleutian Islands. It was known as the "birthplace of the storms." Seems that all the storms headed for the West Coast of the United States start in Adak and head southeast. In one year, I recall only four days of clear skies and little or no wind. The rest of the time it was wind, rain, snow, sleet and an occasional rare glimpse of the sun.

August 22, six months after her marriage, I received a letter from Sara:

> *Sometimes life seems to deal some unbelievable blows and now I'm on the receiving end. Two weeks ago, my husband came home and said he was filing for divorce. All this while — six months — I thought we were a happily adjusted married couple. Boom! The 'star-glazed' world of Sara's suddenly shattered. I'm groping for a friend, perhaps we could write again, that's all up to you. Thanks again Vern. You've always been much too good to me. Hope to hear soon.*
> *Love 'Sam'*

Of course I wrote her back and tried to console her although I admitted I really didn't know what to say.

Her own divorce was almost as traumatic as her parents' divorce when she was a child of about ten. She underwent medical care for awhile. Her divorce was finalized October 27, 1961.

Sara wrote frequently, I guess out of loneliness and despair and needing to tell her story to someone. I would write her cheery letters in return, trying to make her feel a little better by telling her of my dreary existence on Adak.

January of 1962, I received orders transferring me from Adak back to Marine Corps Schools, Quantico, Virginia. My flight from Alaska would land in Seattle.

Early March Sara wrote:

Now I may be stepping way out of line and I'm sure you will understand and tell me the truth. But if you like I would be glad to drive up to Seattle and pick you up. If you like I could bring your mother. It's just a thought and Dad would let me have the car, and my boss would let me have the day off if you arrived on Friday. Anyway it's a thought, and no intention of putting you on the spot. Talk about taking a lot for granted but I must be getting forward in my old age too. I will be waiting with bells on if you want to see me.

Although I was looking forward to seeing Sara, I could still feel a twinge in my heart as I remembered our last two times of being together, and the ending goodbye letters from her. This time though, with Sara taking the initiative, maybe it could work. Maybe indeed the third time would be the charm. So I wrote back and said that would be fine and I would be looking forward to seeing her.

I departed Adak in early March and arrived in Seattle. Sara was there to meet me. She wore a smart gray business dress with black stockings. She had lost weight from her San Francisco days and she looked great!

All my life, I have tried not to rush into hasty decisions. I try to take important decisions "under advisement," which means I think them over and possibly do some research on the subject. But suddenly I decided to make a decision! At twenty-seven, with a rather beautiful twenty-six year old woman right in front of me, I decided that life was not to pass me by. I was going to risk opening my heart again, with all its passion.

I asked Sara to marry me. Now, not later. She said "Yes," rather excitedly.

First things first, I guess. I called Sara's father, Dick, and asked if we could meet for lunch. Dick agreed. We met in downtown Portland, near the Oregon-Washington-California Pear Bureau. Apparently it was one of his favorite places, because everyone knew him. After a couple of drinks with lunch, I quietly informed him that Sara and I were getting married. I don't remember a lot of the conversation, except Dick did say quite emphatically, "I'm not going to pay for another wedding, I just paid for one." I nodded my head to let him know I wasn't here to ask him to do that, I just wanted to marry Sara. He acted relieved, and then told me, "You know Sara needs to be taken care of." I wasn't quite sure at the time I understood what he meant by "taken care of," but I nodded my head and said, "I'll take good care of Sara."

Time was of the essence! I had to be to Quantico on time. Thirty days leave can go in a hurry. So many things had to be done.

First I had to pay for the wedding and make arrangements for us be married at the Portland Air Force Base Chapel. Sara and I had to be interviewed by the base chaplain. He was not particularly happy with the hastiness of this marriage, particularly in view of Sara's recent divorce. As I recall, I told the chaplain in no uncertain terms, "We are getting married and if you do not feel comfortable performing the ceremony, I will find someone else." He agreed to marry us.

Then wedding rings. Sara wanted to use Zells Jewelry in Portland, so we went to have wedding bands made.

It was rather short notice and there was no time to send out formal invitations, so we spent a lot of time on the phone notifying friends and family in the area.

Sara's mother was going to fly in from California. She missed Sara's first wedding in Texas, as her father had paid for that one and they still weren't on the best of terms. She wasn't going to miss this wedding, regardless of the short notice.

I had to find a best man so I asked my brother Don who was living in Portland. Sara found a sorority sister to serve as her maid of honor.

On April 14, 1962, Sara and I were married in Portland, Oregon. After the wedding we packed the gifts we had received into the trunk of my car and took off for a motel in town for the night. The next night we stayed in a motel on the slopes of Mount Hood, and the following day headed east for Quantico, Virginia.

On our trip across the country we talked about our hopes and dreams. Sara told me what she wanted out of life. "A happy marriage, home, and a station wagon full of little children. That's what a woman is for. Some women don't want this, but it's my life's goal."

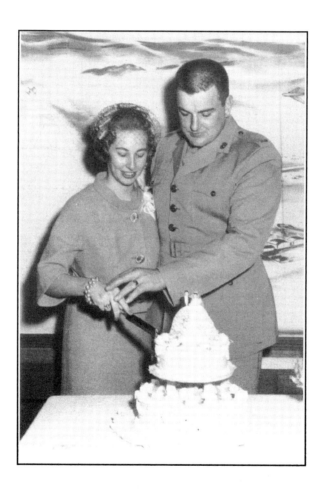

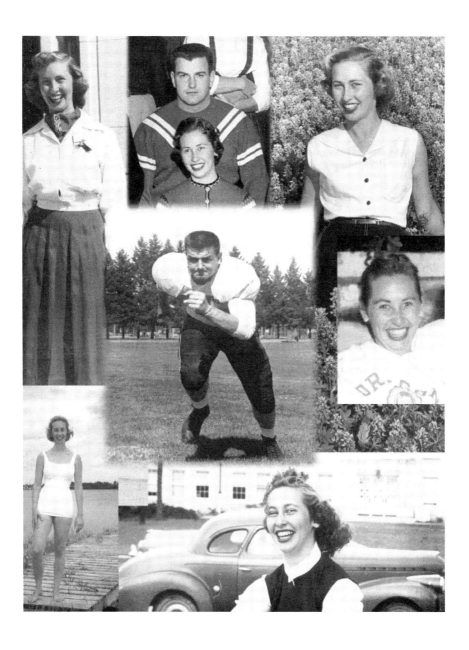

Chapter 3

A Station Wagon Full of Children

S ara had always looked to her father for advice and any real decision making, both as a child and as a young adult. She and her mom talked, but in the end, she went to her father for the final say. Sara told me, "You know whatever Dad suggests seems to be right for me."

After we were married, Sara just transferred that responsibility to me. She looked to me for advice and decision making. Even when I tried to sometimes include her in rather complex problem solving, she shied away. She preferred for me to make the decisions and tell her specifically how she could support me. Many times it appeared to me she was afraid of making mistakes and that may be why she chose the support role.

It was a winning combination for us, whatever the reason. Like her dad, I was a person that felt more comfortable in the decision making role and I could always count on Sara for giving tremendous support.

When we arrived in Quantico, Sara and I found an apartment over a garage in nearby Triangle, Virginia. Sara referred to this as "the tree house." Squirrels were everywhere. I put up a platform in a tree outside the kitchen window, where we would put food out for the squirrels.

Sara went about turning our little house into our home, putting all her Home Economics education to work. She was a fabulous homemaker. A friend of ours gave her a book entitled, *The Marine Corps Wife*, which spelled out guidelines for every possible situation she might encounter. She referred to it often as her "guide book" and I always felt great pride when people complimented on her perfect etiquette within the Marine Corps.

Life was good in the tree house.

As soon as Sara got settled in as a homemaker and a Marine Corps wife, she wanted to start on her next goal — filling up our car with little children. It took about a year before Sara was to become pregnant, only to suffer a miscarriage. She became very depressed and questioned her ability to become a mother. She remembered her own mother's unhappiness over her early attempts to have children. Sara often lamented that she didn't want to be like her mother in this regard. The Quantico Marines football team doctor, a team I helped coach, who was to become a good friend, spent some time counseling Sara over this issue.

Luckily, it wasn't too long before Sara became pregnant again. She was truly elated!

It was on the final night of the All-Marine Corps Basketball Championships, that as athletic director, I had to coordinate the final ceremonies. It was a big night and the Commanding General would be present. Sara found this to be perfect timing by saying, "I think tonight just might be the night that I'll need to go to the hospital." I wasn't able to take care of both commitments, thus I called Ray and Teresa Stephens, friends of ours, to see if they could stand by in case Sara needed to go to the hospital. Teresa said, "I'll be available, but Ray will be there at the basketball game." I asked Sara, as if it were within her power, "Could you try and hold off until later in the evening before delivering?" Sara just looked at me and smiled.

At the basketball game, I got a phone call from Teresa saying, "I brought Sara to the hospital, but there's no baby thus far."

After the championship game was over, the awards presented and the General on his way home, I headed for the hospital. Sara was doing well and had waited for me. At 1:49 a.m. on February 25, 1963, our daughter Darby Ann Ellison was born.

On first viewing Darby, it looked like she had been hit in the head with a hammer. Her skull had big dents in it, but I was informed that's normal, and that they'll go away. They eventually did.

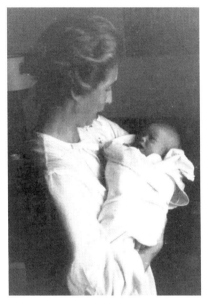

We were both proud parents, but to Sara, it was even more. She felt secure and accepted in her role as a wife and homemaker. Now she was complete in her role as a woman. I had never seen her happier than when I saw her holding Darby close to her heart.

Then just a few months later, as the situation was heating up in Vietnam, Sara became pregnant again. The advisory days were over and we were now committed to the fight in Vietnam. On March 8, 1965, the U. S. Marine Corps moved into Danang. In the winter of 1965, I got my own orders to Vietnam.

We decided the best place for Sara to be while I was in Vietnam was back in Portland, near her father. Dick would be close by, and he could look in on her frequently. Certainly I felt relieved knowing he would really watch over Sara and Darby.

Between apartment hunting in Portland and getting Sara and Darby settled in, we enjoyed a party or two, mainly for the purposes of sending me off to Vietnam.

I was to note some four years later that the same support for the Vietnam War would for the most part be absent. The war was new at the time and not fully understood. As time passed though, the attitude of many Americans changed radically regarding our involvement in Vietnam.

When it was time for me to climb on a train to California and catch my flight to Vietnam, Sara was in her eighth month of pregnancy. Neither of us liked that I had to go, but after all there was a war going on, and I was a Marine.

On arrival in Vietnam, one of the first people I ran into was Ray Stephens. My initial assignment was as the assistant operations officer of the 4th Marine Regiment.

While in Vietnam, Sara and I wrote each other most every day, sometimes more than one letter. We made a conscious effort of keeping our family together, in spite of the war and the distance. However, the mail, at both ends, was not daily delivery of a letter, but usually two, three, four and even five letters all arriving at the same time. I never had any complaints of the mail service while in Vietnam.

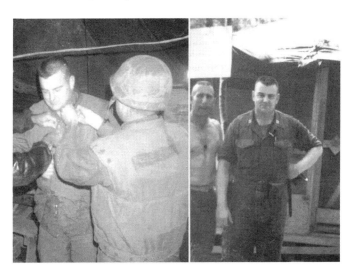

My Dearest Darling,

Because of the airline machinist strike made up my mind it would be a long dry spell not having mail from you. Was so surprised to receive four letters from you written last week. Between us bet we almost fill the box with our letters - some day we will have to sit in our den with glasses of

champagne, after the children are asleep and reread our let-
ters. I think we will have a fun little family with lots of
catching up to do. Sounds like you're really missing old
Sammy too, glad cause I miss you terribly.
    All our Love, Sammy and Sunshine

A few days before Sara was to give birth, her mother flew up from California for the occasion. Sara's mother didn't drive, but then neither did my mother. That put Sara's father on call for the run to the hospital.

The time came and a call was made to Sara's father, who happened to be on the golf course at the time. He rushed home to the apartment to pick up Sara and make the well planned trip to the Emanuel Hospital located across Portland on the Northeast side. The trip was going well until they approached the Steel Bridge over the Willamette River that was designed to lift like an elevator to let ships pass underneath. On this day, the bridge was up, forcing Dick to find an alternate route to the hospital.

Sara wanted so much for me to be included, that she took a tape recorder for the doctor to tape record the delivery room conversations. It was quite evident by the number of times the tape recorder was turned on and off that things were not going well. She had a very difficult time in giving birth and was in labor for many hours. It turns out that our son was in backwards and upside down. Instruments had to be used to turn him for delivery. Finally, Corbin Vernon Ellison was born April 24, 1966 at 9:49 p.m., weighing in at 7 pounds, 15 ounces.

The stress from the difficult birth and my being gone was too much for Sara. She went to the doctor for a checkup and he put her on some tranquilizer medication.

Dearest Sweetheart,

Received two long letters from you yesterday. Read them
while waiting at the Dr.'s office. I'm trying to get along with-
out the pills - the doctor said for you not to worry now and
the pills don't hurt a thing. So very glad I didn't get worse
and made it through a rough spot. Old Sam wouldn't let

you down, sweetheart. Darby is reading your letter now.
She liked the picture you drew for her, and she carried it
around with her all day.

   All our Love, Sam, Sunshine and Corb

Sara's condition distressed me, but there was nothing I could do except to write her even more letters. Even though Sara and the kids lived close to her father, he moved them in with him. He had room now, he had just put his mother into a nursing home, due to senility, because the care for her had proven to be too much for him.

Dick was a great communicator, and kept me up to date on the daily activities in a humorous way. I really enjoyed his letters.

   Dear Vern (When in hell are you going to be
   Major?),

   Everything is well under control. Both kids came up
   with colds and were very generous in spreading them around,
   first, Darby and then Fat Joe (one of Corbin's many nick-
   names), Sara and finally Boompa (Sara's father's nickname).
   They can certainly be crabby when they don't feel well. It
   sort of gets to Sara. She is a great little mother and very
   devoted, but a damn poor disciplinarian. Now that both
   kids are recovering, she is hauling out a blade of grass now
   and then. If you have any grass in Vietnam with blades over
   three inches long, you had better bring a small supply home
   with you. Ha, Ha, that's a big laugh. I can just see you
   beating hell out of those two kids when you get home. I can
   just see one big Marine completing the job that Sara and I
   have so nobly started. We ought to get one thing cleared right
   now. We don't want you unspoiling those two kids - that's an
   order.

   Both are growing like weeds and getting cuter every
   day. Darby is starting to use sentences. She pretty well in-
   forms you as to what she wants. Fat Joe (Corbin) has a rare
   assortment of sounds and gurgles, which Sara somehow in-
   terprets as Ma Ma, but to me it sounds like food, food. He is
   starting to get some coordination in his hands and believe

me, nothing is safe within his reach, not even the table cloth with everything on it. He is strong as hell. I don't believe I've ever seen a happier, little guy in all my life. He's got it.

Now for "Old Vern," I guess I can understand your disappointment in not getting a rifle command. But think about it, how can you win a war without reams and reams of paper? Keep winning the war - stay behind the desk - zig instead of zag - we want you home soon.

As ever, Dick

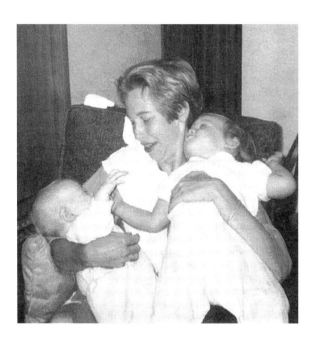

When we got married I am sure Sara couldn't visualize our current situation. She had her hands full, especially with my being away. It was hard on both of us not being together, but for Sara it was more so.

Dearest Vern,

Here's old shakie Sam back again. Hadn't had a pill or needed one till Saturday. Now require two a day again. We're just all sick and things are going to hell around here.

Fuses blew, dryer broke, kids sick. Keep wondering if I'm gonna last till you get home. Most times I'm caught in a private hell of my own.

I shop with tears in my eyes all the time and always in a rush to get outside. God, how I miss you — will these last months ever pass - Old Sam is about the end of the rope. I'm so tired of doing everything about to pop. Got to go as can't keep eyes off Darby one sec. She woke up quite a few times cause of her cold. Little devil wipes and blows her own nose, hard to believe. Thank goodness for small favors. Love you so much, dream of your loving me and so real - tears me up - hardly wait for you, darling. Please come home, hope it's a 12 month tour by some grace of God.
All my love, Sam, Sunshine and Corb

I believed that being away in the service and sacrificing for our country was my duty and I accepted it. As I was growing up, Patriotism, serving in the armed forces, defending our country, and even the world, were high ideals. Now that I was an adult, it was my turn to help ensure that our country and even the world was safe. I didn't question my tour of duty in Vietnam.

Sara was getting reports, as well as I, about the number of divorces and other domestic problems military families were facing as a result of Vietnam. Somehow, probably by staying so connected through our letters, our marriage not only stayed intact but our love grew. Sara had a way of making me feel like I was part of the home, even though thousands of miles away.

Good morning,

The slides came Sat. Funny to see you in glasses - you look very wise!! Also tired. You know it's going to be quite a challenge for you to give both of em all the love, and playing they want. Corb is playing peek-a-boo with me while I write - Darb is talking to your picture. Darby says to tell you "poddy trained" - of course you heard that a 1000 times now but she insists I tell you often. She also says "tell about books." She has a load of books for you to read to her. Sure glad you will be home soon so we can smile all the time. Darby carries the latest picture of you - with glasses - all around. Hope we have a letter today. I anticipate your letters all morning, then cry over them when they come or cry when they don't come - what a dope I am!

All our love!

I was promoted to Major January 16, 1967, with a date of rank of January 1, 1967. The regimental commander and the operations officer pinned my Major leaves on me while standing outside the operations tent in the rain.

Our dearest Daddy,

Your major promotion orders came today in good condition - effective as of 1 Jan. How about that? Will put them in the file cabinet. Couldn't resist putting Major on your letters today as you indicated you have your leaves on as of the 15th. Congratulations. Now if you could only get a good job. You should see Corb play ball - he's a wild man and the ball goes everywhere and he's right after it. He's standing beside me now blowing bubbles. Darb is on the other side cooking. Talk to you later sweetheart - have to feed the dog. Darby's bumping my elbow as I write now.

All our love, Sara, Sunshine and Corb

The many pictures that Sara sent me over the months, just showed how fast little kids grow.

After ten months as the assistant operations officer, and on promotion to Major, I was reassigned as the regimental logistics officer. The Captain, who was my assistant logistics officer, reported that his wife was on tranquilizers also. So Sara was not alone.

At age two, Darby could spell her first name, lace her own shoes, name a whole bunch of birds in her bird book and partially dress herself.

I had received information earlier that I would be transferred to Headquarters, U. S. Marine Corps in Washington, DC and had been expecting orders anytime now. Neither one of us looked forward to returning to the East Coast, but at least it meant we would be back together as a family.

Finally my tour of duty in Vietnam was over, and I was headed back to the states. It was so good for us to be back together again. I spent the first few days getting reacquainted with Darby and meeting my son for the first time. After the children were asleep, we found time to toast each other with glasses of champagne, just like in Sara's letter to me. After celebrating Corbin's first birthday, we were off, driving across the country again to the East Coast.

We bought our first home in Springfield, Virginia just south of Washington, DC.

As expected I was assigned to the Personnel Department and subsequently as the Head, Sports Unit, Special Services Branch, Headquarters, U. S. Marine Corps. My basic duties were to plan the execution of the All-Marine Corps athletic championships in various sports, such as basketball, boxing, softball, golf, tennis, track and field and handball, but I would also be involved with the National Championships and the Olympic movement.

The job was one that would see me traveling almost continuously. Due to the high cost of phone calls, it wouldn't be possible to call home much.

One of my first trips was to Minneapolis, Minnesota for Pan American game trials, and then on to Winnipeg, Canada for the 1967 Pan American Games. Looks like Sara and I would be back to writing letters again.

Dearest Daddy -

We were so glad when your letter came and the funny card. The children really liked seeing where you are staying - pretty snazzy - Darby enjoys your letters and talks about things you say in them. Tonight a big airplane went over and she shouted, "There goes Daddy!" Today was a real busy one - Dr. told me that the birth control pills I'm taking are not foolproof! God, that shocked me. Corb is 16 months old today. Cute little devil. He tries to talk and says so much now. Little Miss Muffet is a real talker too and comes up with real good words. She's 2-1/2 years old today! Have quite

a few surprises around the house for you. You have to come home to find out though. We love and miss you. Keep both feet on the ground like the card you sent.
   All our love, Sam, Sunshine and Corb

Sara and the kids picked me up at Dulles International Airport, something they did many times over the next three years. If not Dulles, it was Washington National. They were always glad when I returned from a trip and I was thrilled to see them after such a long time away.

Sara and her mother kept our children well dressed. It seemed sometimes there was a contest between the two to see who could create and sew the best outfits.

While I was away on another trip, this time to Athens, Greece, Sara decided it was time to improve her cooking skills, and enrolled in a cooking class. Sara always was a very good cook, as were her mother and grandmother. Cooking was one of her favorite household activities. Over the years she built a rather large collection of cookbooks numbering into the dozens.

Our tight budget was brought to the forefront one day, when I came home early and unexpected. As I drove into our driveway and got out of the car, I saw a woman walking out of our front door with a big laundry basket full of clothes. I didn't recognize her. When I went into the house I asked Sara who that woman was. Sara was quite evasive and stammered before she finally explained. Her concern for our lack of money made her decide to earn some of her own. She decided to take in laundry and ironing. For the first time I can remember, Sara had done something that I found rather upsetting. I really couldn't picture the wife of a Major in the U. S. Marine Corps having to take in laundry. As I recall, after a rather short discussion, Sara agreed to stop her laundry business.

It seems the birth control pills she was taking were definitely not foolproof. Sara announced that she was pregnant and expecting March 16, 1970. Everyone was excited with the news, particularly Darby and Corbin.

I was determined to be with Sara this time when our next child was born. I promised Sara. I even turned down a three-week trip to Russia at the end of January. I couldn't take the chance of not being there. Every day Corbin asked her, "When are you going to hatch?"

Sara's due date was March 16, but she felt it might be sooner. On March 13 in an attempt to speed things up, she decided to serve creamed tuna on toast for dinner. She said, "That's what I had the night Darby was born." A fun idea, but it didn't work.

March 15th and still no baby. I caught Sara jogging around in the snow that afternoon in our backyard! Sara was determined, as well as being anxious.

With no noticeable reaction to her jogging, we went to bed as usual. At 12:30 a.m., Sara woke me up excitedly and said, "It's time to go." Our neighbors, a Colonel and his wife, said they would take care of Darby and Corbin, when the time came. Well the time had come, so I called them to come over as I loaded Sara into the car.

The birth of the baby was scheduled for Bethesda Naval Hospital in Maryland. We got on the beltway and headed north from Springfield. There was little traffic at that time of night, so it didn't take long to get to the hospital.

I checked Sara in and proceeded to the waiting area. There were two other men in the waiting room, one of which had two little boys with him. We all just sat and waited.

Finally I heard a squeaking noise, and saw a baby crib being rolled into the waiting area. The nurse asked for Mr. So and So, and the man with the two boys came over to the crib to check out the new addition to the family. Finally they all disappeared. That left the just the other guy and me waiting

Eventually, I heard the squeaking noise again, but didn't pay much attention, until I heard the nurse say, "Mr. Ellison?" My first reaction was to stupidly say, "It's not my turn." Then I realized that although the other guy got here ahead of me, my baby was a little quicker than his was.

I went over to take my first look at Amy Joyce Ellison who was born at 4:03 a.m. on March 16, weighing in at 8 pounds, 4 ounces and measuring 20 1/2 inches. She didn't have the dents in her head like Darby. I was one proud father and especially pleased that I was able to be there when she was born. I hadn't liked it that I wasn't able to be there for my son's birth.

Sara had been apprehensive about delivering because of Corbin's difficult birth. I was worried about Sara and went in to see her. She smiled her wonderful smile and said, "Everything is fine. The delivery turned out to be quite easy, like Darby's." I must say I was grateful and relieved.

On arriving home Darby and Corbin were waiting excitedly. Both of them jumped up and down and wanted to hold Amy, which they both did. Amy was to be the center of attention for some time in the future. She was our last child.

As Sara found out, the pill was not foolproof. Of course, we were glad it wasn't, as we got to have Amy. Now though, we both agreed that it was as much my responsibility as Sara's to ensure that we had no more children than we could take care of, both emotionally and financially. We decided that our family was just right as it was now. So I had a vasectomy.

Raising our children in a way that we could be proud of was the road ahead of us now.

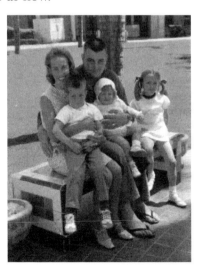

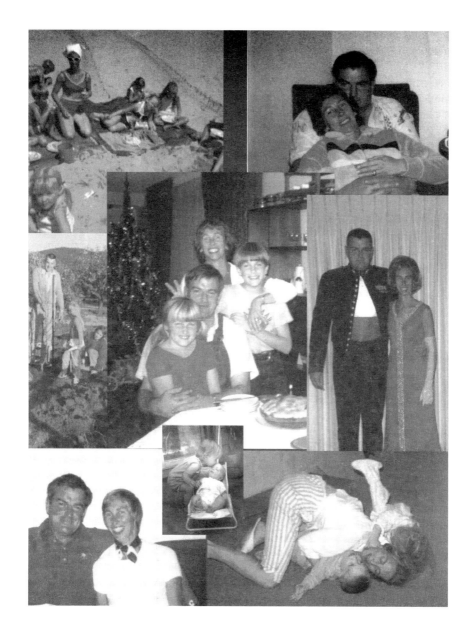

Chapter 4

Sara Excels at Career Goal

Shortly after Amy was born I was transferred to Camp Pendleton, California. Sara couldn't have been more pleased. However, when I reported in for duty, I found out that my orders had been changed. I was headed to Okinawa.

Sara was devastated! There was nothing we could do though. Sara's father had remarried, so moving her back to Oregon didn't seem like an option to us. I did the best I could to care for my family. In Oceanside, near Camp Pendleton, I purchased a new home for Sara and the children. Then I departed for Okinawa.

Once again, I was assigned to special services, which involved athletic and recreation programs for the Marines. Sometimes I wish I had never been a football player in college. No matter what I did, it seemed I was always put into special services. As far as I was concerned, it ruined my career in the Marine Corps.

Sara and I were back to keeping our family together by our daily letter writing. We really missed hearing each other's voice and would have liked to stay in contact by the telephone. However, commercial telephone calls from Okinawa to the States were quite expensive.

Luckily I learned of another alternative. There was a Marine Amateur Radio Station (MARS) available. Under this system, one could place a telephone call via radio to the States. The MARS operator would call another amateur radio operator in the States. That operator would place a telephone call to the party you wanted to call and then patch the radio into the phone line. Thus I would call Sara and we could talk, the only cost was the phone bill between the stateside amateur radio operator's location and that of our home in Oceanside. In this case it was a call from San Bernardino, California to Oceanside.

A necessity in the radio/telephone conversation was the requirement of saying "over" when one person would stop talking, so that the other person could talk. It would be like, "Hello, over." "Yes? How are you? Over." "I am fine, over."

After a few phone calls, we had the system down pretty good to where even Darby and Corbin could say a few "overs."

Sara wrote once:

> *"Let me tell you how much I appreciate you writing to me everyday and finding something interesting to write home about. It really chills me to see how some wives and husbands treat each other. I still wouldn't trade you for anyone else in the world sweetheart."*

She had a point. One of my fellow officers remarked one night it was time to write his weekly letter to his wife. He indicated he only wrote once a week because there was nothing much to write home about.

Besides the letters and MARS telephone calls, we created another way to keep our family together. Sara got a tape recorder, as did I, and we started sending tapes back and forth. The children really enjoyed talking on the tapes.

One morning while shaving, I noticed a bulge on the right side of my neck. I watched it for a few days but it did not go away. In a few weeks, I found myself on a plane headed back to the states for an operation. Aboard the flight to San Diego, I read Sara's latest letter where she reported she was down to 101 pounds and not faring too well. Amy was suffering from constant ear infections topped off with a case of German Measles. Not sure how Amy got German measles and Darby and Corbin didn't. Corbin missed his nursery school's visit to the San Diego Zoo because of an ear infection.

I felt bad for Sara, I knew my health problem would be an additional burden on her. Although I had to be operated on, the bulge turned out to be a benign tumor. Both of us were relieved. Even better, I didn't have to return to Okinawa, but was transferred to Camp Pendleton, just minutes away from our home in Oceanside.

The rest of my military career was spent on the West Coast with my family. We were both healthier and under less stress once we were back together.

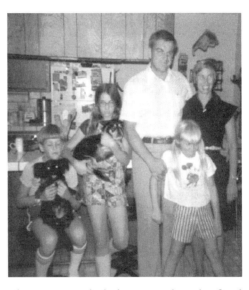

Unless there was conflict, which Sara always deferred to me, on the home front Sara managed the family affairs. She would tell the kids, "Wait until your dad comes home. He'll decide what to do," or "You know your dad always makes the final decision. He'll be home soon."

In 1973 we moved from our tract home in Oceanside to a country home in Vista.

Darby and Corbin both enjoyed their new elementary school, where Sara again was deeply involved. Together, we were active parents with the Parent Teachers Association (PTA).

Our family garden was becoming quite large and I was enjoying growing a wide range of vegetables the year around. Somehow Sara also found time for herself, she rode horses at the base stables and enjoyed tennis at Camp Pendleton.

I was a transferred to the Marine Corps Recruit Depot in San Diego during the summer of 1975. This would be my last assignment.

I would be retiring in June 1977. Fortunately San Diego was close enough that I could commute for my last two years from Vista.

I completed the requirements for a Master of Arts degree in physical education during the summer quarter of 1976. A Masters degree was a requirement if I wanted to try and teach at Palomar College once I was out of the Marine Corps. Sara didn't want to return to Oregon, she was happy with our life in Southern California. I had been working part time since 1971 assisting with the football program and teaching. I felt that was probably the direction our lives would take.

As I approached the end of my career in the Marine Corps I was teaching racquetball a couple of nights a week at Palomar College and was going to be teaching during the summer session as well. May 31, 1977 was my last official workday in the Marine Corps. I would return at the end of June to be officially separated and retired. The general public's attitude toward the armed forces had dramatically changed since I joined twenty years ago. I wasn't sad that my time was up, in fact I was looking forward to it. Sara felt the same, she had never really been happy as a Marine Corps wife, although she never showed it.

I immediately started teaching at Palomar College after leaving the Marine Corps in 1977. My time at home was now quite significant in comparison to the previous years. I had time to take Corbin shooting, which is something I had always wanted my dad to do with me, but he never seemed to have the time.

It became evident in 1978 that our home was becoming a little crowded. Corbin, 12 and Amy, 8, were sharing a room and it was quite evident that a change would have to take place.

On a rainy December day, Sara and I were out driving around and found a For Sale sign on a house in an area that we liked. We called the real estate agent listed on the sign and made an appointment to look at the house. It was a big house, nearly 3,500 square feet on an acre of level land, on Catalina Avenue, in Vista.

There was an old barn, about 20 by 40 feet in size, with a tin roof full of holes, some distance from the house. There were four different species of palm trees, all kinds of fruit trees and a place for a huge garden.

After much thought, Sara and I decided to make an offer to buy the house. This offer involved a lot of financial maneuvering. The offer had to be contingent on selling our present home. It required me to borrow money against two of my life insurance policies.

Sara and I spent the next three years repairing, painting, wallpapering and remodeling inside. Sara got quite good at hanging wallpaper and decorating. Her mother continued to supply us with artwork of all kinds. Her mother's pictures ended up in just about every room in the house. Outside, I worked on turning the horse corrals into a nice large garden. We also added some more fruit trees and removed other trees.

Life was good on Catalina Avenue!

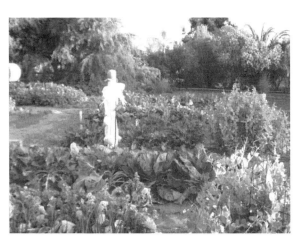

At Palomar I was elected as the athletic director although I still remained as an assistant football coach. I was now involved with all the men's sports: football, basketball, baseball, wrestling, swimming, water polo, tennis, soccer, track and field, cross country and golf. I held the post of athletic director for two years and then decided not to run again.

I could see financial problems ahead with the children about ready to enter college. The next year I would just coach football and teach, then finally just teach. I heard one time that one of three

California residents had a license to sell real estate. I decided I would become one of the three. I had Sara's support in this decision.

In May 1983, along with probably a few hundred others, I took the real estate examination in San Diego. The money from my real estate efforts was timely. Our first child, Darby graduated as one of the top students in her high school class and had been accepted at the University of California at Irvine (UCI). She would major in biology and psychology.

Sara earned a recognition award in 1983 from the Vista Parks and Recreation. I do not recall what the award was for, but might have been in connection with her helping form a woman's tennis club through the Vista Recreation Department. In previous years, she had brought home a couple of tennis trophies from the Vista Parks and Recreation tennis tournaments.

June of 1984 saw our second child, Corbin, graduate with honors from Vista High School. He would be off to the University of California at San Diego (UCSD) to major in biology and anthropology.

For the next few years as Amy was finishing up high school, Sara continued her volunteer work, particularly in support of Amy's participation in the high school band. All through the children's

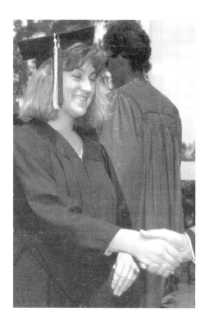

high school experience, Sara would not miss an event. Sara would be there for Darby as a member of the Tall Flag contingent, Corbin in soccer or Amy playing the saxophone in the band. I would attend many of the events myself, particularly if they were at night.

Sara still played tennis almost daily. She started volunteering to drive elderly women from a couple of retirement homes for shopping and doctor appointments. Sara was also involved with the Boys and Girls

Club, Parks and Recreation, the Children's Home Society, Panhellenic and P.E.O. She would never tell me what P.E.O. stood for — I just knew it was a secret. But the organization was basically involved with continuing education for women.

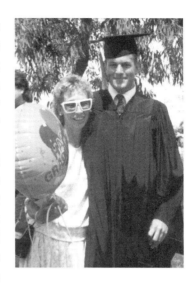

During this period, I continued teaching and working in real estate. We also took time to do things together and enjoy each other. Both our families were important to us, and throughout the years we would take trips to Oregon, as well as to Placerville for visits. In the summers, I would go to Utah fishing, and on occasion Sara would accompany me. We also saw Las Vegas and Laughlin, Nevada on more than one occasion, which we both enjoyed.

Sara and I often talked about our accomplishments both as a couple and in our role as parents. We were really proud of ourselves. With a lot of hard work, we had created a home environment where our children excelled in school, didn't get into drugs, and seemed happy and well adjusted. Also, instead of dwindling, our love and respect for each other kept growing throughout the years.

Without a doubt, Sara had gotten what she told me she had wanted out of life. A happy marriage, a home, and a station wagon full of little children. Not only did she reach her goal, she excelled at it.

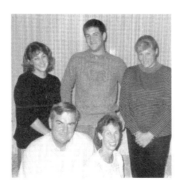

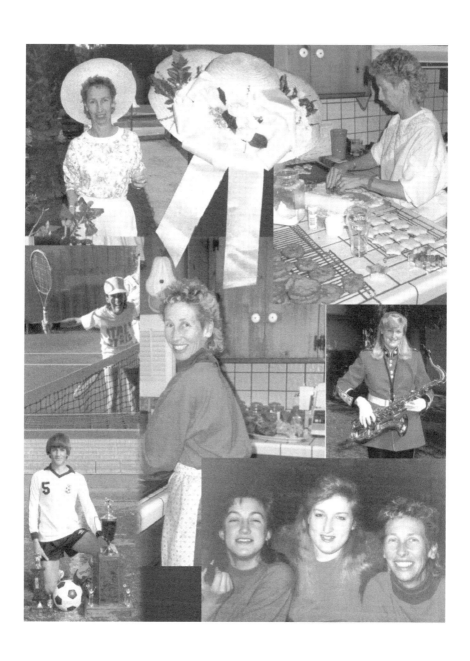

Part Two
Down a Road of
No Return

Chapter 5

Bizarre Behavior

*J*anuary of 1988 our lives swerved off the road we were traveling on, onto a new road from which there was no turning back. Of course we didn't understand that at the time, it's only while looking back that I can get some perspective.

The first time I ever noticed what I would term bizarre behavior was when my mother and sister stopped by for a visit on their way back to Oregon from Arizona. Throughout our entire marriage Sara always made a special point to be very respectful and cordial to my family. She never complained about my family or was critical of them to me. As I've been writing the book, I found letters to her mother and found out from my oldest daughter that Sara did indeed have the normal in law upsets that most families have. Still, to my family members or to myself, you would have never known it. She was always eager to please them.

It seems Sara had set rules that she lived by, and being respectful of my family was one of them. I would find out later

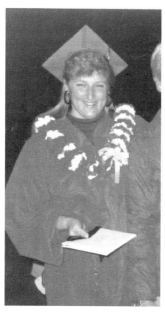

through my daughter Amy, that another of the guidelines Sara lived by and taught our children was "never rock the boat."

This visit was different. Sara was not only disrespectful, but she rocked the boat until it almost overturned. Sara became very hostile and impolite to my mother and Virginia. We were all mystified and maybe even shocked. This was totally unlike Sara. None of us could understand or explain what was happening. Once they left, Sara seemed fine again, so even though I was most upset, I didn't hold a grudge.

Life continued. June 1988 saw our youngest child, Amy, graduate from high school. She enrolled at Long Beach State University to major in criminology.

As Amy was entering Long Beach State, Darby was graduating from the University of California-Irvine. She had no job offerings yet, so she moved back home. As soon as she moved back home, the Bren Events Center at UCI called, offering her a part time job. She commuted for awhile. Then they offered her a fulltime position and she decided to take it, thus moving back to Irvine.

Sara and I were left completely alone now, except for our dogs, Lucy and Spud, and our cat, Spot. The coyotes had gotten Gotcha a few years before.

Sara began to exhibit some signs of depression, such as sadness and loneliness.

Even though she still had her volunteer work, none of it involved her own children. Raising a family had always been Sara's only career goal. Since that time was over, it was as if she had no purpose. She tried to fill up her time with more tennis, but clearly there was a void.

About this time the local newspaper ran an article about a group of women who called themselves "The Big 5." Sara was one of the group written about in the article. The five women had met years before while their children were attending Monte Vista Elementary School. The article told how the five women had volunteered their services in support of their eleven children from grade school through high school. It talked about PTA projects, fundraisers, countless meetings, and cookie baking. I would say the article was about five women who actually practiced what has been termed so often in the 1990s as "family values." The Big 5 continued to meet for luncheons and birthdays well after all the children left high school.

Luckily, Corbin was close enough to drop by frequently and if we wanted to take a short trip somewhere, he would stay over and care for the dogs and cat.

On one such short trip, Sara and I went to Las Vegas for two or three days. A set of bizarre incidents happened during that trip that really puzzled me. Twice while we were in a casino, Sara went off to the bathroom, telling me, "Don't move from that slot machine you're playing until I get back." Both times I was paged over the casino's public address system to go to a certain location to pick Sara up. She said, "I couldn't find you because you moved on me." I hadn't moved either time. I couldn't for the life of me figure out what was going on. Sara was so sure I had moved, yet I knew I hadn't.

Then the night before we were to go home, after dinner Sara suggested, "If you'd like to, why don't you stay out and play cards all night. It's all right with me. I'll drive us home in the morning." That sounded great to me, and I did just that. I stayed up all night, first closing down the seven-card stud game at the Desert Inn and then going across the street to the Frontier and playing until 6:00 a.m.

When I got back to our room Sara was irate. She said, "I've been up all night worrying where you were." When I reminded her that it was her idea, she acted as if she didn't know what I was talking about. She remembered nothing of what she had said, it was a total blank in her mind. I felt totally confused now. First she was sure I had moved in the casino when I had not and now she was sure she hadn't suggested I play cards all night. Needless to say, I drove home, somewhat taken aback by it all. What was going on? That was it though, for when we got home Sara was back to herself.

The next time something strange happened was a couple of years later. For some years, Sara and I had thought about taking longer trips outside the United States. One of them was to Australia and New Zealand. Finally, after extensive research, on December

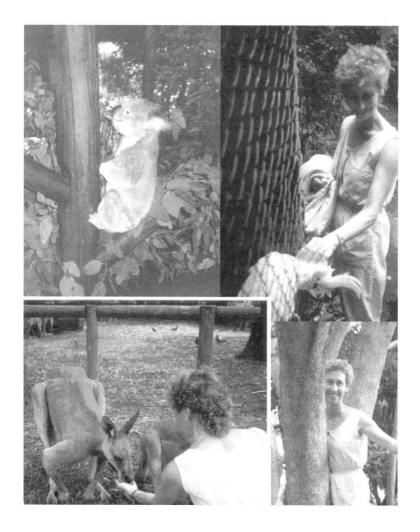

28, 1990, we left from Los Angeles for Australia. We landed in Sydney and took a connecting flight to Brisbane. We rented a car and proceeded to drive south from Brisbane to Melbourne, making planned stops along the way. From Melbourne we flew to Auckland, New Zealand, and again rented a car to drive around the North Island.

We were staying at Lake Taupo. While we were there, the television was reporting that the U.S. had started bombing Iraq.

For some reason during the last three or four days of our trip, Sara became very worried, confused, and outwardly afraid. She couldn't understand the time differences between New Zealand and the United States. She kept worrying about missing our return flight. I kept telling her, "Everything is fine. There's nothing to worry about." Her fixation on missing our flight became almost her only topic of conversation. She kept asking the same questions about the flight over and over.

We made our flight with no problem. However, we were held up in Los Angeles International Airport due to heightened security measures and this caused additional stress. She remarked angrily, "Why is it taking us so long to get through customs? We're American citizens." She became very agitated and vocal.

Sara was changing in front of my eyes from an outwardly happy woman to someone whose emotions were often out of sorts. If she wasn't crying, she was angry. She attributed her mood swings to menopause, but something didn't make sense. She seemed confused about so many things. No matter how many times I told her about the flight, she'd ask the same question over again.

During the same period, Sara began suffering dizzy spells and went to our doctor. Finally, on June 24, she underwent a MRI to try to determine the cause. We thought for sure the MRI would show what was wrong, but it was inconclusive. Eventually the dizzy spells just went away and I thought nothing more about them.

Sara may have continued to think about it though. During an interview for this book with our eldest daughter Darby, she was asked when she first became aware of her mother's condition. She went straight to the time in November 1991 that she came home from Irvine for a visit. Darby recalled that in one of those mother/daughter talks, Sara burst into tears and said, "I have Alzheimer's. I just know it." This was completely unknown to me, but Darby was the family member that most other family members expressed their feelings to, including my own mother and Sara's mother. If you wanted to know how someone really felt, you could count on Darby to know.

Sara's mother came to visit for the holidays in December of 1991. It would turn out to be her last visit to our home. Sara and her mother did not have a good visit. I'm not sure why. Sara just seemed so hostile and unfriendly the whole time her mother was here. It wasn't quite as bad as when my mother and sister had visited some time back, but it certainly wasn't the Sara that I had been accustomed to for over thirty years of marriage. Sara's mother Shirley, or Grammy as the children had named her years ago, was taken aback by Sara's behavior as well. In fact, Grammy went home and took to her canvas. As an artist, she dealt with her emotions the

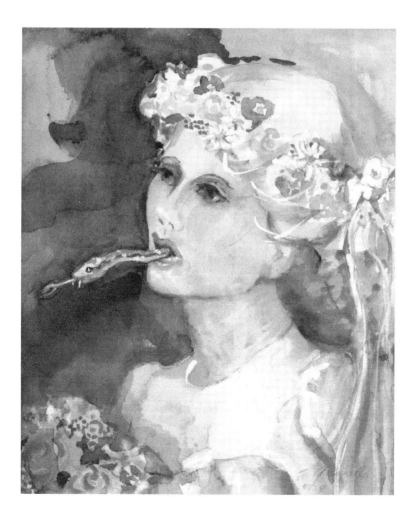

way she knew best. She painted a picture of Sara with a serpent's tongue coming out of her mouth. Underneath the picture, her mother wrote, "King Lear–how sharper than a serpent's tooth."

Early in 1992 I kept hearing, on the radio, an information commercial about a pamphlet on depression available by mail. Some of the things mentioned, such as "diminished ability to think, concentrate, remember things, or make decisions almost every day" and "a sad, depressed, or empty mood most of the day, every day" sure seemed to describe Sara. So I sent away for the information. On receiving it, I sat down with Sara and asked that she read over the pamphlet at her convenience. Later I asked whether she felt she might be experiencing any of the symptoms of depression, especially as it related to memory.

Sara said, "Yes I do feel I have some of the problems mentioned. I have trouble remembering things. And I feel alone and depressed. I'm pretty sure it's because of 'empty nest syndrome' though. With both Darby and Corbin graduated from college and out on their own and Amy still in college, I just feel lonely all the time."

I didn't discount what Sara had to say, but I wasn't so sure this was the only explanation and suggested we talk to our family doctor.

> At this point, to ensure some continuity to the events that are to happen with the medical aspects of this story, and to ensure privacy for all concerned, I have chosen to use fictitious names for those participating in the process.

I suggested an appointment with Dr. Jones, our family practitioner, we had known for some years. Sara agreed, so I made an appointment for both of us to meet with him. We discussed the situation with Dr. Jones. He said he would provide some counseling for Sara to deal with the "empty nest syndrome." At the same time he prescribed a drug called Xanax, which he thought would help her depression.

While we were waiting to see the effects of Sara's counseling and medication, Sara went about her daily life as usual with tennis, Panhellenic, PEO, the Children's Home Society, the Courthouse Children's Waiting Room Program, and her volunteer assistance to senior citizens in a couple of retirement homes. As I drove around Vista in my secondary occupation as a Realtor it was not unusual for me to see her with one or two little old ladies in her car. We would wave to each other and continue on our separate ways.

Corbin was just down the road in San Diego so we saw him often. One day he came home as I was working in the garden, he got out of his pickup and shuffled over to me. He told me he was going to be making a career change, he had been working with the San Diego County Health Department since graduating from UC-San Diego.

I had no idea what he was talking about when he said, "making a career change." Sara and I knew he had been receiving formal letters from various health departments throughout the state, so I figured he was making a move on one of those. What a surprise when he announced he had joined the United States Marine Corps! He was entering the officers candidate school (OCS) at Quantico, Virginia.

Sara was not particularly happy with the news, she was remembering our fifteen years together while I was in the Marine Corps. Neither Sara nor myself had ever tried to persuade or direct any of our children in any one particular direction, except to get the best possible education while they could.

 I was teaching a night racquetball class on Tuesday and Thursday nights At Palomar. On those nights, Sara and I had worked out a simple meal schedule where I would eat leftovers when I got home around 8:00 p.m. One night I came home and she said, "Dinner is ready. Sit down and eat this right now." I was bewildered and said, "No, I'm not ready to eat right now. Remember we have an agreement that I will eat leftovers on Tuesday and Thursday nights." She started yelling, screaming, and swearing at me. As I recall, this was her first real verbal attack on me, but it would not be the last. It was obvious she had been drinking too much, so I gave up and sat down for dinner only to find out she had not even cooked it! This was a really bad night.

Sara and I always sat together when I came home and had one or two cocktails as we discussed our day with each other. It was our way of relaxing and taking some time to be together. Until now, her drinking had never progressed beyond that, except for occasional social gatherings.

I found out later that many people like Sara at this stage begin to drink far too much in an effort to relieve their condition — it's self-medication. Even though I felt her drinking contributed to her behavior, I was also quite sure that it was not the source of her problem.

Sara continued her occasional counseling sessions with Dr. Jones, but unfortunately I could see no improvement in her forgetfulness or depression. She still had difficulty remembering things, although she kept a detailed calendar of things to do and notes to herself about everything. She had always done this, but now she was making mistakes and would white them out and make corrections.

Then for no real reason, except maybe it was intuition, we decided to update our wills, we had written them some time ago. As it turns out, we would need these legal documents later. We also had a Living Will written up at this time. It stated that neither of us wanted our life prolonged by heroic, extraordinary, or costly measures if we could not return to an existence in which we knew what was going on around us.

In Sara's will she was quite adamant about being buried in her tennis uniform with her tennis racquet. It reminded me of one of Sara's posters of a woman of the 1920s era playing tennis. The saying is, "Tennis isn't a matter of life and death–it's more important than that."

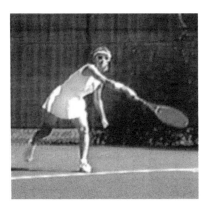

Chapter 6

Nothing Can Be Done

*M*ay of 1992 I received a phone call that was both distressing and hopeful. I was at my office at Palomar College. The call was from one of Sara's doctors, Dr. Black, a gynecologist. Dr. Black started off the conversation by indicating he did not want to alarm me, then asked, "Have you noticed Sara having trouble remembering things?" I not only said, "Yes," but more like, "Hell yes!"

Dr. Black was calling because Sara had shown up at his office for an appointment she didn't have. But what really concerned him was he saw her in his office last month, again for an appointment she didn't have.

We talked for awhile. I explained the concern I had about Sara's depression and that she was presently seeing Dr. Jones, our family practice doctor, for that. After further discussion he felt I should probably refer Sara to a specialist, more specifically a psychiatrist. I said I would contact Dr. Jones regarding our conversation and get back to him.

I called Dr. Jones regarding my conversation with Dr. Black. He had no objection to having Sara referred to a psychiatrist and if Dr. Black had one in mind that would be fine with him. He did ask, as our family doctor, to be kept informed of future developments. I told him I would make sure he received progress reports.

After a few more phone calls with Dr. Black, he recommended that Sara see Dr. Smith, a psychiatrist he had known for several years. I had no objection to his recommendation, I just needed to ensure that our health insurance would cover the doctor he suggested. When I checked with our insurance carrier and I found that Dr. Smith was an approved medical provider, which allowed us to go ahead.

Sara was cooperative during this time and followed along with what the doctors, or I, suggested. She wanted to feel better and eliminate the problems she was having.

We had committed to attend the 35th reunion of my Marine Corps officer's basic school class. The reunion was to be held both in Washington, DC, and Quantico, Virginia. We decided to make a week long trip of it by visiting my brother Don's oldest son and family who lived in the Quantico area.

June 14, a few days before the reunion, we left for the DC area. During our pre-reunion visit with my nephew Richard and his wife Carole, we went for a lengthy ride on the Potomac River in their boat. To make a day of it, we went south and over to the Maryland Shore to a famous seafood place where we had an early dinner of shrimp and crabs.

We had a great time, particularly Sara who loved the boat ride, which made me happy about our decision to take the trip. However, on the way back north the wind picked up and before long we were forced to fight rather large waves coming south right into us. Before long, we were soaked and I was somewhat concerned for our safety. Richard and Carole were not doing a lot of laughing. It was rough. Sara seemed oblivious to the whole thing, as if she were away somewhere in her own world. Of course it was quite a relief that she was not hostile or upset, but at the same time her lack of response was totally inappropriate to the situation. Later I found out this is called "the flattening effect." It took us forever to get back — not until after dark, with an empty gas tank.

The reunion went well and Sara had a great time seeing old friends from our Marine Corps era. Everything was going well until the end and the trip home. There was supposed to have been a function on Sunday that was canceled at the last minute. We missed the notification that was sent by mail because we left several days early. Sara had packed a special dress for the Sunday event. When she found out it had been canceled she just lost it. She yelled, "What am I going to do with the dress that I brought special for the event!" I told her we would just take it back home with us. That did not satisfy her. The tirade went on for some time. I felt distressed, as there was nothing I could do about it. My concern for Sara was growing because once she started a tirade, she couldn't seem to stop until she wore herself out.

Finally we got aboard the plane and headed home. While on the plane, the stewardess came by and asked, "What would you like to drink?" Sara replied, "What do you have?" When the stewardess started to list the usual drinks Sara didn't seem to grasp what she was saying she just had a blank stare on her face. The stewardess kept waiting for Sara to choose and when she didn't, proceeded to tell her every drink they stocked on the plane. At the end, Sara just seemed confused, and she turned to me and asked, "What should I have?" I'm sure the stewardess must have been as frustrated as I was, but I was learning there was nothing that could be done in situations like these.

Upon arriving home, we had to turn right around and plan for a trip to Oregon. My mother was going to celebrate her 80th birthday on the weekend of July 4th. This time we got ready to hit the highway instead of taking planes. We took off for Oregon on June 30, stopping on the way to see Sara's mother in Placerville.

The trip was going fine until we approached Corvallis, just before driving across the Willamette River, Sara announced, "I'm not going to have a good time." It was a prophecy that she made come true. She acted like a spoiled child all the while we were there. She irritated everyone, which was mostly my family, with constant criticism, complaints, and pouting. My brother Don got so mad at Sara he yelled at her, "Why did you even come?"

My mother compassionately remarked, "Sara has changed so much." Mom had always loved Sara as did my father and all my family. So when my mother remarked how much Sara had changed, I knew that Sara's behavior was obvious to most anyone. I had somehow gotten used to her behavior and probably didn't notice it as much as someone who was not continually around her.

While in Corvallis, we took my mother for a drive some forty miles to the Pacific Coast. We stopped on the way at the myrtlewood shop in Philomath. Sara found a small myrtlewood stamp holder, the kind you put a roll of stamps in for dispensing. When Sara tried to charge it on her Visa card the clerk said, "We don't accept credit cards." Sara reacted by exploding. She screamed, "Let's get out of here, they don't want to sell us anything." Mother didn't say anything and was patient while I tried to calm Sara down as I paid cash for the item. I must admit, I became upset, even though I tried not to show it. It was becoming harder not to show my concern and upset in situations like these. I just couldn't understand what was happening to my Sara, and I felt powerless to do anything about it. Her hostile behavior was increasing all the time, as well as her deep depression.

The trip home was also quite a challenge. Every time we stopped to get something to eat or for gas, Sara would use the restroom. Each time she would say emphatically, "Don't leave me!" It was as if she were becoming paranoid. She acted sincerely frightened. All I could do was to say over and over, "I promise you I will not drive off and leave you. I'll be right here."

We finally made it home to Vista. In late July we had our first appointment with the psychiatrist, Dr. Smith. He started the visit with a conversation about he and Dr. Black being old friends. He told us he had talked to Dr. Black about Sara and the problems she was having. Sara had been seeing Dr. Black for several years and she seemed quite at ease with Dr. Smith, particularly since he was a good friend of Dr. Black's.

I called and talked to Dr. Smith on the phone prior to this first visit and provided him with my observations of Sara over the past few days, weeks and months.

It was decided that Sara would attend, on her own, a series of appointments with Dr. Smith both for counseling and a certain amount of testing.

As this proceeded, so did Corbin's progress in the Marine Corps. It was time for us to take another trip to the East Coast, this time for Corbin's commissioning in the United States Marine Corps. August 14th was the day. As a retired Marine Corps officer, I had the privilege of swearing in my son as a Second Lieutenant. Of course I was quite apprehensive about taking a trip with Sara, but after all this was an important event in our son's life. I know it would be important to him for us to be there.

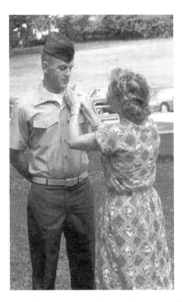

We attended the graduation ceremonies and parade, and afterward I swore Corbin in and gave him my personal Marine Corps officer's sword, purchased in 1957, as a commissioning gift. My name is engraved on the sword and now his is too.

We picked Corbin up at a designated time and place and together headed to Dulles International Airport for the flight back to California. We checked in and proceeded to wait to board our flight. As we sat there, it was announced that our flight was over-booked and the airline was looking for passengers to give up their seats for all those wonderful benefits an airline has to offer for over-booking. Well Sara took that as a threat and panicked saying, "We are going to lose our seats!" She became very loud and vocal saying, "I will not give up my seat!"

Sara became so hostile and irritated in front of the other passengers that Corbin got up and walked away. This was the first time that I knew of where Sara's often bizarre behavior had become obvious in front of Corbin. I'm sure he could see other changes in his mother although we never discussed it. Finally I managed to quiet her down.

Then I heard Sara say, "Don't we know that man?" Where she was pointing I saw the familiar face of a retired Marine Corps Lieutenant Colonel Oliver North, who had been prominent in the news. Sara loudly said something like, "Someone will probably blow up the plane." Fortunately, those sitting around us ignored her. I could only say to myself, could it get it any worse than this? Yes it could, and did.

When we got home I decided it was time to brief Corbin on what was happening with his mother. Maybe then he could better understand the behavior he witnessed at the airport. I tried to bring him up to date the best I could. Corbin didn't say anything, although he listened quite intently. Corbin, like myself, often does not express himself with a lot of words.

The fall of 1992 would see Sara carry on with her usual activities of tennis and volunteer driving for her senior friends. However, in September, after nearly a year with the Courthouse Children's Waiting Room Program, Sara resigned. This resignation was apparently over some confusion and disagreements with the program leadership. Poor Sara, now her condition was becoming obvious in her volunteer programs also. I wondered how long it would be before she wouldn't be welcome anywhere, even as a volunteer. Sara kept reporting people were yelling at her all the time. They were probably just trying to explain to her what to do and she was too confused.

On October 20, Sara renewed her California driver's license through the mail. Later this was to become a major problem for her both mentally and emotionally.

In November, Sara volunteered as a "cuddler" for newborn babies at the local hospital. She would work two, four hour shifts each week. It was a job she loved and one that she seemed able to do.

Sara was subjected to testing under Dr. Smith's direction. This involved a referral to Dr. Brown, a neurologist. Now we had a family doctor, a psychiatrist, and a neurologist attending to Sara. I just hoped that between all of them, they could find out what was happening to my dear Sara.

Dr. Brown began his own independent evaluation of Sara. We had good insurance, which absorbed most of the costs.

At this stage, I went with Sara to all of her appointments as I felt I needed to know what was going on. I felt I could probably remember the facts better than Sara could as she was becoming more and more confused. After consulting with both of us, the neurologist ordered a MRI and brain scan, both of which were conducted in late November. The test results were sent to our psychiatrist who showed me, but not Sara, the results of the test. He told me that he found there were some irregularities in the brain and it was in a state of deterioration. He said, "There is nothing that can be done about it." I don't think I even reacted to what the psychiatrist was saying. I just felt numb as he said those dreadful words, "There is nothing that can be done about it."

Dr. White was becoming involved in the process, she was a licensed psychologist who was trying to discover the exact cause of Sara's behavioral changes. She conducted a battery of tests on Sara, which resulted in a long, written evaluation of the results. It would take me weeks to obtain the written results, but Dr. White shared the results early on with both Dr. Smith, the psychiatrist and Dr. Brown, the neurologist.

> Whatever the cause, I had to come to grips with the fact that Sara's brain was deteriorating and nothing, but nothing, could be done about it. I think that was the beginning of my own depression. I began to feel sad and empty most of the time, myself.

Sara was also visiting a chiropractor, Dr. Bendher, fairly often. Off and on over the years Sara had suffered back problems, possibly due to her tennis activity or maybe my bowling class, in which she continued to participate during the fall semester at Palomar.

With great pride I remember one of Sara's earlier achievements when my insurance had denied coverage of her chiropractic treatment. It was clearly unfair and Sara and Dr. Bendher took the insurance carrier to court. Sara had to stand up and present her arguments before the judge. She won her case and the insurance carrier had to pay. I was there to watch the proceedings and must admit Sara did a wonderful job presenting her case.

In remembering the old Sara, it made me sad to realize that if Sara had to do the same thing today, she could never present her case, much less remember much of it. It would just be a waking nightmare. Poor Sara, what was I to do? I must admit I was beginning to lose hope — and if I was losing hope, I could only imagine how it felt to Sara. Needless to say, these were all private thoughts that I never discussed with Sara. I always wanted to sound hopeful to Sara.

I continued teaching at Palomar along with a variety of other activities, but started cutting back my involvement in real estate. I was on the Board of Directors for the California Community College Association (CCA) and every month or so I would have to fly off somewhere, usually to San Francisco, for a weekend meeting.

Sara was still heavily involved with tennis at our local park facility and was down there early almost every morning.

Darby and Amy came home for Thanksgiving. Darby was still working at the Bren Events Center at the University of California-Irvine and Amy was nearing graduation from Long Beach State University. Corbin enjoyed Thanksgiving dinner at his cousin Richard's house just a few minutes from the basic school at Quantico. As the test results were not all in yet, I decided not to discuss the neurologist reports with the kids. I didn't want to alarm them any more than necessary.

After the holidays, I sat down to pay our monthly bills. I had been in charge of finances all throughout our marriage. Sara had a few minor bills she would pay. Together we had a joint checking account and Sara had her own private bank account. I thought about the day I would probably have to close these accounts, but right now I just couldn't bring myself to do that.

Christmas came and the family all made it home, including Corbin. Sara and the girls pitched in to cook a nice Christmas dinner. For just a few moments, it felt we were a normal, happy family enjoying Christmas together. Instead of being happy though, I found myself feeling somewhat sad knowing what lay ahead. I wondered if this would be our last Christmas dinner with any semblance of normalcy.

Chapter 7

Once Turned On,
Can't Turn Off

*T*he year of 1993 started off with some hope of getting to the bottom of Sara's condition. In the first week of the year, Sara and I met with Dr. Brown, the neurologist, to go over the full test results. Now Sara would hear for herself what the psychiatrist had already told me earlier. I decided it would be best if Sara heard directly from a doctor instead of me, in case she had any questions that I couldn't answer. Besides I couldn't bring myself to tell Sara that there was nothing that could be done for her condition. I was still struggling with the facts myself.

I watched for her reaction as Dr. Brown told us that she had irregular patterns in her brain and it was in a state of deterioration. There was no reaction from Sara, not even a question. She just accepted what was said almost as if she wasn't a part of what was being discussed. Dr. Brown did not put a label on Sara's condition or offer a diagnosis. He just went over the test results.

A meeting followed this appointment between Sara and Dr. White, the psychologist, for further evaluation. Dr. White did not give a diagnosis either. It had been over seven months now since our doctor, Dr. Black, called me at work to ask if I might have noticed Sara not remembering things, and I had said, "Hell yes!" I remember being so glad that someone had noticed what I had been living with.

We had been through seven months of testing, including physical examinations, neurological tests, mental status assessments, analyses of blood and urine, CAT scans, and a MRI. After all the meetings with the psychiatrist, psychologist, and now the neurologist, not one doctor would, or could, come out with a conclusive diagnosis. It looked to me like they were in a process of ruling out what her condition was not, as clearly, not one single clinical test could pinpoint Sara's condition.

The testing was hard on the nerves, especially as Sara's condition kept worsening. Sara was becoming disoriented and unable to do many things for herself. She was trying so hard now to keep her life together, but her calendar book was really a representation of what was happening in her mind. The notes and calendar she kept were in a constant state of flux at this point. Her use of Liquid Paper correction fluid had become rather dramatic as she changed her calendar, then changed it back, and then changed it again.

Dr. Brown, the neurologist, had basically taken over Sara's case, although he kept in contact with Dr. Smith and Dr. White. My hopes for counseling sessions helping Sara with her depression were gone. All signs were leading to the conclusion that Sara's problem was physical, specifically with her brain.

Finally, in early February, Sara and I had an appointment with the psychiatrist Dr. Smith. During this appointment Dr. Smith verbally discussed Dr. White's findings with us. Again Sara had no reaction, either in his office or later after we went home.

He gave us a copy of Dr. White's report to take home. Dr. White's report was replete with medical terms I did not understand. Her findings were written more for doctors than for a person like myself.

I looked up one word after another in a medical dictionary until I could understand the report. I was determined to fully understand what was wrong with my Sara. There were however, some comments that I could understand all too easily.

*****

Summary of Report Contents

At the time of this evaluation Mrs. Ellison demonstrated a range of neuropsychological functioning from average to severely impaired.

Most notably her long term memory for both verbal and visual information was quite severely impaired. New learning was very slow and memory for everyday behaviors was severely impaired.

These test findings suggest a significant decline in several neuropsychological functions when compared to expected functioning for the client's age, gender, and educational background.

The following recommendations are offered as coping strategies to enhance Mrs. Ellison's functioning:

1. Stick to a daily routine and minimize disruptions/change.

2. Anticipate changes and alterations of daily routine.

3. Control the client's anxiety to enhance her ability to think clearly without the paralyzing effects of anxiety. Pharmacological and/or behavioral methods may be useful, depending upon the client's response.

4. Similarly, improvement in the client's frustration tolerance would maximize her functioning, and reduce the likelihood of oppositional behavior and refusal.

5. Acquire the habit of writing down information for later reference. For this the client will need some assistance or reminding to recognize which information is important for later use. It is recommended she carry a note pad in her purse.

6. Use visual cues around the home such as signs, labels, markers, etc. to identify important information. (For example: turn a clean/dirty sign on the dishwasher, note the upcoming time to leave the house by the use of a clock sign with movable hands.)

7. Do not rely upon the client's memory. Anticipate that she is apt to forget factual information, particularly information that changes often such as dates, times, sequences, and multistep information. Do not expect her to retain new information without many repetitions.

8. When possible provide associations to help the client to remember. Do not "crowd" her memory with unessential information, but rather have her try to remember things of greater relevance and personal need using natural association to things already known.

9. Provide both auditory and visual input of information. Write down instructions or develop pictures/signs which depict the information to be remembered. Use as many different sensory inputs as possible.

10. Important information is best remembered with frequent repetition of input and practice in recalling, although there should be no pressure upon the client to remember information.

Because of the client's difficulty in cognition her adaptive and coping resources are significantly compromised. As such, the burden of adaptation and accommodation falls primarily to Mr. Ellison, who must learn to manage their lives in light of the client's difficulties.

Mrs. Ellison is not a good candidate for individual therapy due to her poor learning, memory, and loss of mental flexibility, which make significant behavioral change difficult. However, family therapy is recommended for this couple to devise methods of reducing the client's anxiety, providing support to Mr. Ellison, and increasing the client's self awareness and acknowledgment of her difficulties so compensatory strategies are used.

Mrs. Ellison's cooperation must be enhanced and her defensiveness decreased, while Mr. Ellison must recognize ways to avoid frustrations for both he and his wife. Clearly Mrs. Ellison readily becomes defiant and accusatory when frustrated, which only exacerbates the problem. Family therapy may be helpful to address this pattern of reaction and identify a less stressful interactive style for this couple.

Lastly, repeat neuropsychological evaluation is warranted in twelve to eighteen months, or when warranted by change in the clinical status, to assess any change or developments in the client's cognitive functioning.

*****

At last I had something in writing that gave a very detailed analysis of Sara's condition. The diagnosis was pre-senile dementia. The word Alzheimer's was never mentioned.

As I began to understand the medical report, I did not discuss it further with Sara. First I don't believe she would have comprehended it, and if she did, it might have thrown her further into depression. I didn't want to hurt Sara in any way. Two different doctors had told her now what was wrong with her, and neither time did she ask any questions or have any reaction. I didn't think my discussing it with her would be of any help. I knew that I could help Sara follow the recommendations that were made — most of which I was already doing.

Based on all the evidence thus far assembled, Dr. Brown, the neurologist, informed me that by law he had to notify the Department of Motor Vehicles (DMV) of Sara's apparent status. I asked, "What does that mean?" He said, "As a matter of policy, she must be reexamined to determine if she will still be allowed to drive."

There was not much I could say — I just wish Dr. Brown had told her and not left it up to me. But then he didn't often see us together. The children had all remarked that Sara had been unwilling to drive on the freeways or major highways. For a few years now Sara had been taking side streets to get wherever she wanted to go.

I really didn't know how to break this to Sara. Finally I informed Sara that Dr. Brown said she would probably have to retake her driver's license test. She told me that she had just renewed her driver's license by mail in October, which I already knew. I didn't try to explain it to her, I knew that would not work. I just tried my best to let her know without being too alarming. I told her we would just have to wait and see.

Sara continued to manage life the best she could and I tried to assist the best I could, while not acting like I was trying to interfere. It was quite a balancing act that wasn't always possible. Her ability to perform routine tasks was rapidly deteriorating. She had been a bank teller before we were married and loved numbers. Now when I went to the checkbook, I found she had entered the same deposit twice.

She left the water running while watering plants and flooded our street. Her disorientation was worsening, almost as if she was losing her connection with her mind, which I had to remind myself was what dementia was.

Corbin was to graduate from the officers basic school in March and I didn't even discuss going back for the ceremony. The trip would just have been too much for Sara. Luckily, his orders had him transferred to the Marine Corps Base at Twenty-nine Palms, California, so he would be just a short drive away. This made us quite happy.

In March, only two months after Sara started in the hospital auxiliary, she had to quit. Supposedly it was over a disagreement with leadership, which meant to me that she was too confused to follow directions. It was sad to see the volunteer jobs she loved doing all throughout our marriage coming to an end. She even had to quit the job cuddling newborn babies, which had become her easiest and favorite volunteer service.

May 4th, there was a new development. Upon returning home from an evening racquetball class I witnessed what I was starting to refer to as a "memory blackout." Sara would do and say things that later she would not remember. On this date, Corbin had come home to attend a funeral. He told Sara he did not know when he would be back home and not to fix him any dinner. But she went ahead and cooked him a dinner anyway, impatiently waiting for him to return. He did not return until after Sara had gone to bed, and got up and left before she got up.

While waiting that night for Corbin, Sara talked to me about the subject of the DMV notification. The notices I told her about earlier had arrived. She received not one, but two notices regarding being reexamined for her driver's license. Sara had been reading them, which I must admit were a little confusing. She was upset and kept talking about already having had her license renewed in October. As calmly as I could, I just repeated that due to her recent medical experiences she would have to be retested.

I explained the first letter to her and clarified what was to happen. The second letter was confusing, so I called the DMV for clarification. Afterward, I typed a note to her and explained as clearly as I could how things were to be done. More and more I was putting things in writing because when I spoke to her she couldn't grasp what I was saying. The note seemed clear to her. She acted as if she understood. It was a dead issue, I thought.

But that night she read the note I wrote her over and over again. She concentrated on the part about being reevaluated through a telephone interview with a representative of the DMV. She got into a state of total confusion and asked me the same question over and over again. I tried to answer her from every possible perspective, but nothing worked. It was like a switch had been turned on and couldn't be turned off.

I finally said, "Please stop." She said, "You're putting me down. All I've done is ask you a simple question." Sara didn't realize she had asked the same question over and over with only seconds or a minute between repetitions. I could find no way to turn off the switch. I asked her again to stop and said we could talk about it later.

At this point she became outraged and started yelling things like: "You are a shithead!". . . "All you do is put me down when I ask a simple question!". . . "Why don't you just pack your bags and get out of here!". . . "If I had a gun I would shoot you!". . . "If I had a gun I would shoot myself!". . . "Why don't you just kill me and get it over with!". . . "I'll just take the car out and wreck it and get it over with!"

And after all of that, she took a breath and asked me the same question over again about the driver's test. I almost lost it, it was all I could do to hold my own feelings in check.

During this confrontation I told her to please write down her complaints about how I've treated her and how she feels about me, then we could discuss them with Dr. Smith. I realized we needed help, although I wasn't sure he could help us. I doubted she could even remember what happened tonight.

I slept very little. It was that night that I decided to start keeping notes, a semblance of a diary, some for my own sanity and if the doctors needed a full report, I would have it. I started carrying 3x5 cards in my pocket so I could record events as they occurred. I could now see a very long road ahead and where it was going I did not know.

When I awoke at 6:30 a.m. the following morning, Sara was quite cheerful. As always she appeared to remember absolutely nothing about the nightmare of the previous evening. She told me once again about her eye examination from yesterday, the same report she had given me the night before when I came home.

I reminded her that I would like her to write down all of the concerns she expressed last night so she could discuss them with Dr. Smith. She looked at me as if she were wondering, "What are you talking about?" She definitely blacked out after these episodes, I'm sure in part due to the amount of alcohol she was drinking, but that wasn't all of it. She just said, "Everything is fine."

These episodes were occurring too often as of late. Last night I felt like I would become physically sick. I knew the DMV situation had her feeling very stressed. She had never had an accident in over thirty years of driving and she wondered, "Why are they after me?" A feeling of paranoia accompanied her words.

It was getting to the point that I felt like I was walking in a mine field every time I came home from work. I never knew what was going to set her off. When something did set her off I couldn't stop her until she became physically exhausted. Every morning she would get up, the sun was shining and all was fine again. Only I, remembered the horror of the night before.

Chapter 8

She Can't Remember,
I Can't Forget

*S*ome days are pretty good, but then some are just a living nightmare. I am getting very tired. The crying, threats, yelling and swearing just wear me out. In over thirty years of marriage, I can't recall Sara ever once swearing. Now she is doing it all the time.

I guess the big problem for me is Sara can't remember and I can't forget. Not a good mix.

Corbin has been living with us for a short time while he's still in the Marine Corps. He is aware of the deteriorating situation with his mother and tries to make the best of it. Sara cooks much more for him than he can eat. Pies, cakes, lasagna and then gets concerned when he doesn't eat it all. He asked her to cut back, but she doesn't understand. As time went along Corbin began to notice that many of the ingredients in the recipes were left out, giving rather peculiar tastes to the meals. Sometimes they weren't even cooked.

We continued our joint counseling sessions with Dr. Smith. Sara is being medicated for her hostility. The term "sun downing" is introduced, but Alzheimer's is still not a term used. We're told dementia patients seem to become more hostile in the late afternoons and early evenings, when the sun is going down, thus the term.

May 20 was to be another tremendously bad day. Sara washed and dried clothes. Unfortunately, she washed one of my shirts that had a ballpoint pen in the pocket.

She washed the shirt, but when drying it in the dryer, the black ink ruined several items of clothing and some new towels. Sara just lost it. Over and over she told me she did not know what had happened. Over and over I tried to explain that simply one of my ballpoint pens had gotten washed and when drying it got ink on all the clothes. My explanation, as usual, was not satisfactorily assimilated into her thought processes.

I was leaving in the morning for a CCA meeting in Oxnard, I told Sara I would take her with me and for the past two weeks she had been thanking me for letting her come with me. She acted so scared about being left home alone and was glad to be going with me.

But now things had changed with the "stroke of pen." Sara said, "I'm going to buy a new washer and dryer this weekend. All the clothes and new towels are ruined!" I kept telling her the problem was over, gone, the problem was not the washer and dryer, but the pen. Then she just flipped out.

> "I am not going with you this weekend, I am going to buy a new washer and dryer!" . . . "I am not staying at home!" . . . "I am leaving and going to my mother's!" . . . "You are full of shit!" . . . "I am leaving!"

It goes on and on. I tell her, "Write me a note telling me that you are not going with me to the CCA meeting in Oxnard." She did.

I am thinking at this time I should inform our neighbors of our situation, but I have a suspicion they suspect something already.

In the morning, I packed and left for Palomar, ready to leave for Oxnard after my last class. Sara called me later saying, "I want to go to Oxnard with you." I said nothing about the night before or her note to me telling me she wasn't going with me. I just said, "That's fine. I'll stop by home and pick you up." Sara had to spend most of her time by herself, as I was in meetings most of the time. I tried to keep my attention on the meeting but I must admit I was worried about what was happening with Sara. She really seemed to have a good time though.

May 26, was Amy's graduation from Long Beach State. Sara, Darby and I, along with Amy's boyfriend and future husband, Marc, would be there. Corbin was training at White Sands, New Mexico and would be unable to attend.

We went up the day before and got a motel near the campus. That night at the motel, Sara lost it again. She screamed, "Get me out of this motel. I want to go stay with Amy." She yelled and screamed at me. She packed her bag and wanted me to take her to Amy's, but I couldn't do that to Amy. She tried to call Amy, but couldn't figure out how to dial out of the room and I didn't help her. She finally threw the phone at me, and missed. Exhausted and crying she went to bed.

Amy's graduation ceremony was held on a bright sunny morning. I brought our camcorder to record the event, but when I tried to use it, Sara would get mad. I have no idea why.

After the ceremony, while Amy was turning in her cap and gown, Sara said with a hostile voice, "I want to go home, pack my bags and go to my mother's in Placerville." Amy, Darby and Marc all witnessed this behavior and were kind of dumbstruck by it all. Of course it was not familiar to them, they hadn't had to go through almost a daily routine of it.

We finally got in our car and headed home. Sara said, "I want you to leave. I want a divorce." We discussed the concept of a separation and divorce. She said that is what she wanted. Here I was with the woman I loved, losing her a little each day. It seemed there was nothing I could do. When I tried to do what I thought was right, it would be wrong.

In the morning, for once Sara has not forgotten. She writes up questions on how a divorce could be handled.

On May 28, I attended the Palomar College graduation ceremonies. I came home and went right to bed. I was exhausted.

The next evening, I went to play poker at a nearby poker club. I have been playing poker off and on over the past few years. It's something I have to concentrate on and gives me some relief. On returning home I found a couple of notes in the kitchen from Sara.

> *"Vern–No divorce no separation–just as usual–you play cards when you want to and this (is) best for you! I love you–Sara."*
>
> *"Vern–I promise I will not aggravate you ever–I love you! Sara."*

In the morning I got up. I heard Sara from the living room saying in a confused voice, "What happened?" I went into the living room. A lamp had been knocked over and the shade was broken, a world globe that had been sitting on a plastic stand was knocked over and broken, the VCR on top of the TV was pushed up against the wall, the power was on and the video door was open. One of the connections in back of the VCR was bent and another disconnected.

I had purchased a voice activated tape recorder to help me validate Sara's moments of forgetfulness and often I would play back things she had said the day or night before, even minutes before, only to find out she couldn't recall or remember saying what was clear on the tape. So, I listened to the tape from the night before to try and distinguish what happened after I had gone to play poker. I could hear Sara setting her drink glass down in a glass plate and I could hear her crying. Then there was a big crash. I checked the liquor and it was quite evident that she had kept drinking after dinner and after I left. Sara said, with frustration, "I have a large bruise on my left shoulder and a small bump on my forehead." Sara acted very confused and remembered nothing, saying, "I have no idea what happened."

We went to the commissary at Camp Pendleton after a movie. As we got ready to leave I bought Sara a Snapple ice tea. When we got home, she had not finished her ice tea. I noted that she kept drinking it, but now it was no longer tea. She had put vodka and tonic in the Snapple bottle.

> I'm starting to get really concerned now about her physical safety. How can I watch her twenty-

four hours a day? I have to sleep at night so I can work, yet Sara's restless at night and stays up for hours alone.

I got a call in my office at Palomar College on June 1st. It was Dr. Bendher, Sara's chiropractor, who had treated Sara for the past three or four years. She said she was calling in confidence about Sara. She said, "Sara was at my office this morning and was very rude to my staff. She was upset, confused and angry. This is not the first time Sara has acted like this. Sara used to be gentle, friendly, smiling and soft spoken." Dr. Bendher continued, "I've noticed a change in Sara the last few visits and tried to talk to Sara in private, but she wouldn't speak with me in private." I told Dr. Bendher what Sara had been going through the last several months and what was being done. I told her that I would talk to Sara and see if I could do any good, even though I knew I couldn't. Sara might not even remember what happened at the doctor's office.

While swimming that evening I noticed that Sara had another bruise on the back of her right arm. She said, "I don't know how I got it."

When Corbin came home that evening, Sara had an apple pie and big casserole of lasagna waiting. I talked to Corbin about it. He is having as much difficulty with the situation as I am. As soon as he finishes eating one apple pie, she immediately cooks him another. He said with frustration, "I just can't eat everything Mom is cooking for me."

The next day Sara visits Dr. Bendher. The doctor called me after the visit. She said, "Sara accused me of unprofessional conduct and said that she was going to write to the AMA and report me. Sara said, 'I want my records to take with me.'" Dr. Bendher told me that she told Sara it would take some time to make copies and why not sit down and rest before leaving. Sara finally left without her records.

That evening Sara said nothing about her visit to Dr. Bendher. She did say, "I feel that swimming will take care of my back problem and have no need to see a chiropractor anymore." I didn't say anything, I just listened.

Sara kept crossing off friend after friend and didn't even know it. She kept saying people were yelling at her, being rude and impolite. I am sure they all tried to reason with her on some issue and she just couldn't understand, and thus they lost their patience with her. Sara has, or did have, many friends in tennis, clubs and activities, but I saw them dropping away.

On June 4, Sara was to be retested for her driver's license. She drove to the DMV office in her car. I rode with her. As far as I could tell, her driving was just fine. On arrival we checked in and were told that Sara had to take, not a written examination, but an actual driving test. I was told, "You cannot accompany your wife with the DMV employee while she is being tested." So Sara and the examiner took off in Sara's car and were gone for nearly an hour.

I did not notice they had returned to the DMV office, until I saw the examiner walking into the building. I looked for Sara and asked, "How did the driving test go?" She said, "The only thing the examiner said was that I had not entered the freeway from an on-ramp with enough speed." I looked around for the examiner, but couldn't find her, so we left. We never heard from the DMV and Sara still had her driver's license.

On June 6, we went to the movies. On the way home, without warning Sara asked me, "Do you think I'm getting any better?" I don't recall what I said, I do know I had a big urge to cry.

She thinks she is getting better, but she isn't.

When we got home, there was a phone message for Sara regarding a Panellenic Club matter. I guess I found out for the first time that she was the club treasurer and was being asked to provide a check for $250 for the Rancho Buena Vista Scholarship Fund. She was very confused over the request, so I called the woman who left the message. We went over what needed to be done and I tried to explain it to Sara. Her memory retention would last less than ten seconds. After much discussion, I informed the woman, "I believe it is in everyone's best interest that Sara resign her position as treasurer." Sara agreed to resign.

> I am getting to the point where I have to concentrate on trying to keep from shaking. I sometimes feel like I am going to get physically sick. Sara feels the medication that Dr. Smith has prescribed for her is working, but I see no benefit.

On June 7, I note that Sara has worn the same clothes four days in a row. The "old" Sara would change clothes two and three times each day. She used to be very conscious of her dress, but now she seems to have her own uniform to wear each day.

Sara's mother was to celebrate her 80th birthday on June 14. We planned to go to Placerville and meet Sara's half brother, John, and his wife, Martha Lou. On June 11 we packed up and headed north. We discussed the trip and decided to drive up Highway 395 east of the Sierra Mountains, to Lake Tahoe where we would spend the night, and then go on to Placerville.

We stopped in Lonepine for lunch. While waiting to be served, I asked Sara where she might like to stay in Lake Tahoe. She "lost it." She started crying, saying, "We are going to my mother's and aren't going to stop in Tahoe." I immediately recognized a no-win situation and said, "Okay we will just keep driving to Placerville." She kept repeating herself. I finally grabbed a napkin from the table and wrote in big block letters "WE ARE NOT STOPPING IN TAHOE." I placed it in front of her and every time she started to repeat herself I would point to the napkin. After a couple of more outbursts, she finally got the message.

With a change in plans, I called ahead to Placerville to make motel reservations for one night earlier than planned.

As we drove into Tahoe, Sara said, "Why don't we stop and pull a few slots?" I looked at her in disbelief for a moment, but then realized she probably didn't even remember her earlier tirade. I just said, "Okay." We stopped and Sara had a wonderful time.

After a couple of hours, we drove on to Placerville to Sara's mother's home. I left Sara with her mother and I went on to check us into the motel and get unpacked. When I returned to Sara's mother's home, Sara had another outburst of anger. In front of her mother, she said, "Vern is a shithead and I will not go back to the motel with him because he will beat the hell out of me." Neither one of us could get her to stop her ranting. After awhile she settled down and I finally got her in the car and to the motel.

In the morning we went to her mother's to wait for her brother and his wife. Sara's mother was in her bedroom, I heard a crashing noise. Sara's mother had fallen over an electrical cord while making her bed. She suffered a broken femur just above her artificial knee replacement. I called the paramedics who came and transported her to the emergency room. During the whole event, Sara did not seem in the least bit concerned.

We were all supposed to go out for dinner that night. After Sara's mother was settled in the hospital, she told us, "Go ahead and have a good evening." Surprisingly enough, we did just that, we had a good evening.

On Sunday, we had a sort of birthday party in the hospital. It was evident that there was nothing we could accomplish, particularly with Sara's erratic behavior. I decide it is best to take Sara and head home. We all said goodbye. We went back to the motel, checked out and started another trip home. Seems like every trip that Sara and I had taken recently, whether Australia, Las Vegas, Oregon, the east coast, have all been some sort of disaster.

On the drive south, Sara begins to question,
"What day is it? What's the date?" It has been a
problem for her ever since we left Vista. She's asked the
day and date over and over and I know my patience is
beginning to give out. In a closed car, there is no way to
get away from her constant questioning.

I was rather upset with it all and guess that is why I wasn't paying too much attention to the highway and my speed. I was going down Interstate 5, toward Los Angeles and I saw a red light behind me, the highway patrol was waving me over. I looked down and saw I was doing 75 m.p.h. in a 55 m.p.h. zone. Just what I needed. I asked Sara, "Please do not say anything." Sara informed me, "I can say anything I want to." I asked her again, "Please do not say anything." Luckily she didn't. I got the ticket from the officer via Sara's window. All the time Sara is nodding yes. At least she didn't say anything. When we got home, I went straight to bed. It had been another exhausting trip.

Chapter 9

Let a Car Kill Me

On June 15, Dr. Jones prescribed Xanax for me to take as I saw necessary. I didn't like the idea at all, but I told him I'd give it a try. I also picked up a new prescription for Sara, called Tranxene, prescribed by Dr. Smith. Sara's new medication worked perfectly for two days. Sara lost it the third day over a pizza I was picking up for Corbin. I had my tape recorder ready to go, so I turned it on.

> She calls me a "shithead" again, which seems to be her favorite, as of late. She also told me, "Pack your bags and get out of here. I want a divorce." Finally, I left and went to play poker. In the morning, Sara remembers nothing and asks, "Why is there leftover pizza in the refrigerator?" I play back the tape from last night. She remembers nothing.

She kept saying, "You're going to beat the hell out of me." Yet I have never hit her in my life. I remember she wrote about her first husband beating her up and almost killing her. I wondered if she was beginning to confuse us.

On Monday, June 21, when Corbin got home from work, he asked me about Sara's behavior. Apparently the previous night when I was out playing poker, Sara had started yelling and crying. She told Corbin, "I hate your dad and am going to live with Amy." Then she told him she was going to leave and go live with her mother and even with her father, who had been dead for many years. Corbin was very upset over the whole thing. I tried to explain the situation his mother had been going through the past few months and even years. I decided to talk to Corbin about Sara's first marriage, especially about Sara saying he nearly killed her, but I found out he never knew about it. Darby knew, and I just assumed Corbin did too.

After dinner, Sara started arguing again. I went into the living room to watch TV and try to avoid another yelling session. As I was sitting watching TV, Sara walked over and hit me in the face. Unfortunately, Corbin walked in just as she did it. She walked back into the kitchen, only to return in a few minutes. She asked me, "What happened to your face?" It turns out she cut my face, as she hit me, with her ring. I was bleeding and hadn't noticed it.

On Tuesday, Amy came home for the night. Sara had written down that she was coming, but then had forgotten. I discussed Sara's situation with Amy as I had with Corbin. I talked to Amy about Sara's first marriage and found out she had never known about it either.

Sara played tennis Wednesday morning, but came home early. She said, "I left early because some woman started yelling at me." I took this to mean that Sara had gotten confused and made a scene of some kind.

Amy left in the afternoon, saying that she and Sara had had a good day together. After Amy left, Sara lost it again. She started crying and making threatening physical moves against me. She said, "Pack your bags and get out. You are a son of a bitch and I am going to live with Amy, Amy said I could." Between the crying and yelling, Sara says, "I'm so lonely without the kids. I'm really sad."

More and more Sara becomes remorseful. She
is always angry now, not just every once in a while,
but consistently. She says, "I don't know why I'm so
upset all the time now. Maybe it's just because I
miss the kids." How I wish I could somehow help
her, but all my efforts are met with hostility.

In just a few years, Sara has gradually changed from a very
nice, relatively happy person to a very unhappy, unpredictable,
unapproachable and hostile wife.

Her present medication does not seem to be working at all,
and her self-medicating with liquor was increasing.

At about 4:30 p.m., I was in the swimming pool and Sara was
sitting in one of the chairs when Corbin came home. He said, "I'm
going over to some of our friends for dinner." Then he left. I had
steaks to barbecue and Sara became very angry that Corbin was
not going to be home for dinner. I tried to calm her down saying,
"It's no big deal." She turned and threw her drink in my face and
went into the house. I got out of the pool and went in the house. I
found Sara on the phone. She called our friends and was angrily
saying, "What right do you have inviting Corbin to dinner and
ruining ours?" She hung up the phone and continued to make salad.
I found this whole thing very upsetting. It was one thing to talk to
me that way, but now to do the same thing to our friends? Like an
idiot, I asked her, "Why did you do that?"

She just turned and threw the salad at me and was getting
ready to throw the bowl when I grabbed her. She said, "I'm going
to call the police." I said, "Fine, call them but I am leaving." Which
I did. I forget what I did, but I had to cool off. I didn't come home
until 1:00 a.m. and went to bed.

In the morning I made a call to Dr. Smith, telling him I had
to see him right away. I met with him and went over the recent
events. He changed Sara's medication to Haloperidol. He said,
"Have her take it at 5:00 p.m. each day. Hopefully it will control
the sun downing effect, and remove all alcohol out of the house." I
agreed. Dr. Smith was aware that we had plans to take a cruise to
Alaska and attend my high school reunion the last part of July and

early August. He said, "The way things are going, I'm not so sure you should try and make that trip." The way our trips had been for some time, I could see his point, but we would wait and see.

When I got home, Sara told me, "I called Dr. Smith and told him that you had been beating me up. Dr. Smith told me that you have new medication for me." She apparently did not know that I had met with him today.

The following morning, while Sara was playing tennis, I removed all the alcohol out of the house except for a couple of near empty bottles, hoping that would prevent an immediate argument.

That evening we were invited to attend happy hour with a friend at a popular North County restaurant. I did not think it would be a good idea, but Sara wanted to go, so rather than cause a problem, we went. When we sat down with our friend he asked Sara, "How are things going?" Sara responded, "Fine except for this shithead. I want a divorce." Our friend was struck dumb and so was I. I don't know why, as I am to the point where I usually can't be surprised by what Sara says. Later Corbin and another couple joined us.

As I was driving home, Sara just turned in her seat and started kicking me with both feet, saying, "Go ahead, kill us." I locked the doors because it looked like she might try to get out while we were moving. Not sure how I got home. Corbin was there when we got home and I told him what had happened and said I just couldn't spend the night at home. I left and got a motel room.

I got home at about noon the next day. Sara asked, "Where have you been?" It didn't bother her that I was not home last night.

Later in the day I called our friend we had been with the previous evening. He said he had watched Sara continuously during the evening and she was different, she looked angry and not the usual happy, laughing person he had known for years. I decided to tell him about Sara's condition. Little by little our friends were finding out first-hand about Sara.

On June 27, Sara left early to play tennis. She left a note about going to the movies when she got home as long as I don't cause any problems. Not sure what she meant by me causing problems? The movie was to start at 12:30 p.m., but she was ready to leave at

11:30 a.m. and wanted to go. So rather than cause a problem, we left and I drove as slow as I could. We still got there thirty minutes early. I bought the tickets and we went inside. I got some popcorn and proceeded to the theater where we were told, "It's not ready yet, we're still cleaning." Sara turned and said, "We're getting out of here, if we can't get seats, why stay around?" I said, "How can we plan on going to Alaska, if a little wait here is going to cause such a problem?" A couple of minutes later the usher let us in the theater.

The movie, *Life With Mikey*, was quite funny, but Sara never made a sound. At the end she said, "I liked it." Not one single expression was visible and even the tone of her voice was just flat.

That night Sara saved dinner for Corbin, who had been to the beach. When he got home he said he wasn't having dinner and said he had told Sara that. Sara once again became angry with me, and said, "I just want out of this world." She said, "No one tells me anything." Corbin later said, "I told mother several times I would not be home for dinner." I told him, "From now on, put any information in writing, then give it to her. Don't expect her to remember what you have to say." He agreed.

Later in the evening I saw Sara once again counting each tablet of Haloperidol in the container. She has been doing this continuously for the last couple of days and it really disturbs me. She keeps saying she does not have enough for the Alaskan trip because there is no refill. Thus she wants to get a refill on the Tranxene, because she has another refill for it. I keep trying to tell her that she is no longer to use Tranxene and that Dr. Smith wants her to use only the Haloperidol instead. I am trying to get her to throw away the Tranxene container, but she won't, and if I do, it will cause a problem.

Sara is all packed for the Alaskan trip, which isn't for three more weeks. When I say packed, I mean she has all her pills ready to go. She said, "Dr. Smith will help us decide about making the trip." I told her, "He's concerned about us making the trip when you keep telling him that I beat you up all the time, that you are scared to death of me and that as late as last Friday, that you wanted a divorce." I told her, "I believe Dr. Smith is worried that I pose a threat to you on such a trip." Sara's response, "Well we will talk to Dr. Smith and he will help us work it out."

On June 28, we met with Dr. Smith again. He met alone with Sara first. When she came out she said defiantly, "Dr. Smith said we could go on the Alaska cruise as long as I don't drink any beer, wine or alcohol." Dr. Smith overheard her say that and shook his head and told her, "No, not until I talk to Mr. Ellison."

After the appointment we went downstairs to the in-house pharmacy to get her prescription for Haloperidol filled. The pharmacist said it couldn't be filled now, it's too soon and we would have to wait until July 19, just before leaving for the Alaska cruise. Sara was upset and confused because the doctor had given her the prescription. I got it straightened out with the pharmacy.

As we left the pharmacy, Sara said, "Go back upstairs and see Dr. Smith." I said, "Dr. Smith doesn't want to see me anymore today. We have another appointment next week." She became incensed and grabbed me and said, "Get back up there and see the doctor." To prevent a scene, I went back up to see Dr. Smith and told the receptionist the problem. She went in to see Dr. Smith and returned saying, "The doctor does not want to see you again today." Sara was upset, but it seemed to satisfy her and we left.

After the appointment, we went to lunch in Carlsbad. On the way, Sara talked about how terrible she was feeling. She said, "I just want to kill myself and get it over with." Like always I tried to find out what she thought her problem was, and she said the same thing she usually did, "All the kids are gone and I'm lonely. Plus I'm going through the change of life." She never once said anything about her dementia or brain deterioration. Sometimes I wondered if she even understood her condition. To Sara the cause was always the empty nest syndrome and the change of life.

When we got to the restaurant we ordered fish and chips. When it was served I said, "Be careful, it's hot. Let it cool down first." Sara just ignored me and took a big bite and burned her lip. She reacted instantly by getting mad and threatened to throw everything on the floor. In a loud voice she said, "I might as well take a bottle of pills and a bottle of booze and just finish myself off." She finally calmed down and managed to finish the lunch and get out with minimal disturbance, except in the eyes of a couple of waitresses.

As we were waiting to cross the street to go to the car, Sara said with total exasperation, "I feel like walking out in the street and letting a car kill me. I want to get it over with." It's not even after sundown, it's early in the day. I am already shaking inside, scared of what the rest of the day will bring.

Chapter 10

I'm Sorry

Sara keeps asking for a drink, although her
prescription of Haloperidol clearly says, "No alcohol."
Dr. Smith was nice enough to write a nice
note telling Sara that she cannot drink any
alcohol, but Sara still asks.

I went next door to visit with one of our neighbors
that evening. They had a party a couple of nights
before, and some of their guests had parked along
our driveway. Sara had gone out and put notes on their windshields
telling them they were parking on our property. I apologized to
them. I didn't want them to think badly of Sara, I decided to confide
in them that Sara was suffering from pre-senile dementia. Although
the doctors had never used the word Alzheimer's I had come to my
own conclusion that Sara was probably in the early stages of
Alzheimer's. I told my neighbors my suspicions.

My neighbors, Lon and Mary Anne Miller, were quite
sympathetic with our plight. Mary Anne shared with me the story

of her own mother who had died of Alzheimer's. The only conclusive way to be sure someone had Alzheimer's is after they die, through an autopsy. That's probably one of the reasons that Sara's doctors have been so hesitant to use the word Alzheimer's. Mary Anne's family had an autopsy of their mother's brain conducted at the University of California - San Diego research center.

The Miller's told me the heart wrenching story of what their family had gone through with the mother. They tried to take care of her mother, as long as they could, at home, with custodial care. Finally they had to institutionalize her in a nursing home. They told me about the mother's memory loss and hostility. They were totally surprised, as a family, when the mother started attacking the father for no apparent reason. It was the attacks that got them to seek medical help. Up until then they just thought it was old age. In hindsight they found several episodes of unusual behavior besides the attacks that could attribute to the disease.

I thanked them profusely for the conversation and all the information. I felt I got more out of the story of their own experience than I previously had with any of the doctors. The medical reports were not enough to educate me on what to expect. I must say it made me feel better about Sara's attacks on me. I couldn't help from feeling that sometimes Sara was attacking me because of something that I had done to hurt her. It was really good for me to hear that Mary Anne's mother also attacked her father for no apparent reason. I went back home feeling more relieved and uplifted than I had in months.

A lot of what they pointed out, I had already gone through many times and their story let me know what to expect in the future.

When I got back to the house, I found three notes from Sara:

Speak to Dr. Smith–perhaps cruise problems will work out."

"We will discuss this with Dr. Smith."

"Vern–I'm sorry I lost my temper with you. I will be a better wife. Love Sara."

The next few days were quite calm. Finally the medication seemed to be working. It gave me some hope. I never did follow through taking the pills for depression that the doctor gave me. After taking one, I decided that I just didn't want to take the chance of becoming addicted to medical drugs.

July 8, Sara called Dr. Smith. She said, "I'm dizzy." She told me he said, "Take the Haloperidol tablets twice each day, once in the morning and once in the evening at bedtime." Leaving nothing to chance, I confirmed this with Dr. Smith myself.

July 9-10th, I had to attend a CCA meeting in Burlingame. I returned late in the evening. The next morning I noticed an empty wine bottle in our glass recycling container. I knew I had to confront Sara with the bottle if I were to help her. At the same time, I knew any confrontation could send her into a rage, which she wouldn't be able to stop until she became exhausted. Still I couldn't see any way around it. The doctor didn't live with us, she was no longer a candidate for counseling, so it was up to Sara and myself to get through this one together.

I took a deep breath, picked up the bottle and held it up in front of her as I asked, "Where did this bottle come from?" She became defensive and said, "I found it and got rid of it like Dr. Smith said to do." I then asked her, "Did you pour it down the sink like you saw me do with the other bottles?" Sara, obviously very flustered, answered, "Yes." I may never know what the truth was. What seemed important was for me to try to help her stop if indeed she was unable to do so by herself.

Dr. Smith requested, "If possible, please set up a meeting for me with your three children." I let him know that I would try to arrange it around our children's schedules. On July 15, Darby, Corbin and I met with Dr. Smith. Amy could not make it from Long Beach.

Dr. Smith went over Sara's case with the children and his concern about her continual accusations that I was always beating her up. He said, "Under the worst circumstances, this could cause legal problems with law enforcement officials." He further expounded, "Sara is severely impaired mentally and is operating at the level of a four-and-a-half year old. The medication should eventually help control her outbursts of anger. It's a question of finding the right dosages of the right medication to fit her needs."

Dr. Smith informed me, "I think it would be a good idea for your children to prepare written statements to have on file, if needed. I would like them to give a description of the interaction they observed directly between Sara and yourself." Corbin had already prepared his statement and Darby would later write one and mail it to Dr. Smith.

Corbin's statement:

To Whom it May Concern:

My mother, Sara Ellison has not been acting normal lately. She has no short-term memory. She sometimes even has trouble remembering what day it is. She is easily con-fused and has wide mood swings. Often, when she drinks or forgets to take her medicine, she becomes very violent to-ward my father, George Ellison. She complains that he 'beats the hell out of her' all the time. She often says that he 'gave her a bloody nose.' Every time she says these things there isn't a mark on her. I've never seen or known my father to hit my mother. However, I have on several occasions seen my mother hit my father hard enough to draw blood. The worst thing is she never remembers what she has done the next morning. She only remembers that she is sorry about something and would like to make up.

Sincerely,
Corbin Ellison

Darby's statement:

Over the past few years, my mother Sara Ellison, has developed memory problems. She also becomes confused, and perception of reality is often different from that of others around her. For instance, she often says the people "yell" at her. It is my observation that she claims people yell at her, when in actuality, they are contradicting her or trying to help her do something a different way.

I have seen her fly into rages for no apparent reason. During these tantrums she claims that everyone hates her, that we think she's not a good mother, etc. My brother has witnessed her attacking my father although I have not seen this.

Sometimes when I visit, she will show me bruises she gets from playing tennis (which she plays almost daily). However, when I make a move to go home, she will burst into tears and claim that my father is beating her. I have never seen my father hit my mother or yell at her. In fact, I am surprised at how patient he is with her, considering that she can be very trying. When she gets very upset, he will often leave the house so that she can calm down.

Since her new medication started, she seems to be calmer and does not have rages or become violent as far as I can tell. Still, the memory problems remain.

Darby Ellison

July 20, Sara met with Dr. Smith who once again told her, "Make sure you do not drink on the Alaska trip." He had been telling her this for some time, but this morning, he said it once again.

This trip is the one thing that Sara has shown real excitement about doing, so if it were possible, I wanted to take it.

> I am very apprehensive about this trip, because every trip we have been on for a long time has been a disaster. We have planned this one for a long time. I know it could very well be our last trip ever. I just don't want to dampen Sara's spirits. I'm glad Dr. Smith told her she could go if she wouldn't drink. Of course Sara promised Dr. Smith that she would follow his orders.

July 22, we started our trip. We stopped in Placerville to see Sara's mother who had been released from the hospital a couple of weeks earlier. So far, so good, there was no incident with her mother. Then we went to Corvallis to see my family and eventually to Vancouver, British Columbia to catch the cruise ship.

For the most part Sara did fairly well on the cruise. She indeed did not have even one drink as far as I know, and since she wouldn't go anywhere without me, I was quite confident she didn't. She did have problems with a couple of bus tours while in port. She became paranoid that the buses were going to leave us stranded and the ship would leave without us. It took some time to get her calmed down, but eventually she did. Another time, Sara couldn't figure out how to work the camera so she threw it to the ground in anger. She never wanted to leave our cabin, except to go to the hot tub

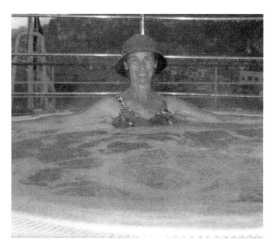

that was on our deck close to our room. At meals she wouldn't talk, which was probably best. Our room was A181, but every time we walked back to our room we had to pass A151. She initially would stop at that door. Each time I would tell her that was not our room, but it made no difference. Transposing numbers was something she had been doing for some time now. To her A151 was the same as A181.

When we got back to Vancouver and were getting ready to leave the ship, Sara became confused and upset seeing passengers leave before us. She couldn't understand that we had to wait our turn. Eventually our turn came and Sara's upset subsided.

We made it back to Corvallis and checked into our motel. The next day, August 2, we were going over to the coast to spend a couple of days. My sister, Virginia, was letting us stay in a beach house that she had. The days were beautiful on the coast, clear sunny skies, which is unusual. Sara was confused about our plans. Knowing that times, dates and days are now always confusing for Sara, I wrote down on 3x5 cards the day, date and what we were going to be doing. Writing them down also helps me. Each time she asks me about something, I can refer her to the cards, instead of having to repeat over and over. It's a lot easier on my own nerves this way.

The following day we drove north to the Tillamook Cheese factory. She enjoyed the drive, but was continually worried about the time and getting back to the beach house.

The next day we headed back to Corvallis and checked back into the motel. Sara wanted to have her hair done, so I made an appointment for her on Saturday.

> At least I'm not surprised when she wants to know the time, day and date of her appointment over and over. The cards help some, but not fully. Finally I say, "Sara, don't worry about your appointment. Leave it to me. I'll take you when it's time." That seemed to work, at least this time.

We spent the next couple of days visiting family and friends. We met up with one of my high school friends and fraternity brother at OSU, and his wife, who was Sara's sorority sister. Before we met, I told them of Sara's condition so they would not be shocked.

Each time I tell someone now, I'm surprised to hear that a member of their family or someone they know had Alzheimer's. Sara's sorority sister told me, "My father died of the complications of Alzheimer's." I also learned one of the parents of another high school friend from Corvallis had also died of Alzheimer's. At least they understood. The real question was how could it happen to Sara? They understood their parents, but Sara was the same age as they were, still in her fifties.

I got Sara to her hair appointment and she came out of the shop looking quite beautiful. Later we went to my high school's 35th reunion dinner. Not once was there an embarrassing incident. Even better, she seemed to have a very good time.

On Sunday there was a barbecue as part of our reunion. I dropped Sara off at her cousin's for the day, while I attended the barbecue by myself. Sara's cousin, Doug Stennett, was a professor in the pharmacy department at OSU and his wife was a nurse who worked in a nursing home with Alzheimer's patients. Both were very cognizant of Alzheimer's, so there was not much I had to say. She apparently had a pleasant day with them. I likewise, for just a few hours I didn't have to worry about Sara. I found myself laughing and talking about some of the good memories in my life.

We went back the same way we had come and again stopped in Placerville to see Sara's mother. The entire trip home Sara asked, "What day is today? How long will it take to get home?" Every time we would get in the car, the questions would begin again. After a very short visit with Sara's mother, Sara said, "I'm ready to leave." Sara's mother, Grammy, said, "I just can't believe the changes I'm seeing in my daughter. She always used to smile, laugh and was friendly to everyone. I just can't believe it's my daughter who's now so angry and always confused."

Finally the trip was over and we made it back home to Vista. One of the first things I had to do was balance our checkbook. I found Sara had entered the same deposit twice. Thinking back on the trip, of Sara's constant confusion with numbers, dates, and times, I shouldn't have been surprised. This was the second time she had done this. Even though I knew full well that I needed to do something with our finances, I put it off again.

We met with Dr. Smith and I reported on our trip. Sara acted as normal as she could. It was a quiet, uneventful meeting.

August 18 was a date and event I will never forget! During the past spring and summer, I had taken the time to prune all of our twenty or so citrus trees. I hadn't done it in a few years, and put in an effort to do a good job, which I did.

This morning I had gone to Palomar College to do some things in preparation for the fall semester. I had a 3:00 p.m. appointment regarding real estate. On my way to my appointment, I stopped home at 2:30 p.m. to see how Sara was doing. I couldn't comprehend, as I drove down my driveway, what I was seeing. There was a truck and trailer in my driveway. I could see branches of trees being loaded into the truck and trailer. I saw several people moving around my house and trees. I just couldn't figure out what was going on.

I pulled in my driveway, got out and started yelling frantically, "Who the hell are you? What are you doing?"

I am incensed! There were five guys chopping away at my trees, the very ones that I had taken so much pride in caring for myself. Finally, the person in charge made himself known. He said, "I came by yesterday and talked to Mrs. Ellison. She hired us to have all the trees trimmed, in front and back."

I couldn't believe it! This included all the trees I had just finished doing, plus the dry root trees, which are pruned only during the dormant season.

I can barely control my anger as I listen to him. He said, "Mrs. Ellison had signed a contract to pay $2,500 to do the job." He showed me the contract and indeed Sara had signed it.

Sara was gone when I arrived. Then she drove in the driveway. I frantically asked her, "What have you done?" She said, "I told them not to do it. It was too much money." The man in charge protested, saying "Mrs. Ellison gave me a check for $100 to start the job." I told him, "Pack up and get out of here. My wife is not well. She was wrong in hiring you. I will give you $500 if you will leave right now and get off my property." He nodded, and I wrote him the check. He took it, loaded up and took off.

I'm sure I asked Sara in a tone of voice that was indeed accusing, "Where do you think we have $2,500 to pay for a job that was not needed?" Sara acted like she had no idea what she had done or the financial commitment she had made. Sara's effort to explain didn't make any sense even though she tried several different times to explain. What she said was totally confusing. All I could think of was that I was lucky I decided to stop home when I did. I might have ended up in jail if I had arrived later and my trees had been damaged any more. There would have been no way I could have kept control of my anger.

There's no way I can ignore now that Sara can do us great financial harm. I'm not sure what to do about it. Finally I went out and bought a couple of "No Soliciting" signs to post. I put one in the yard and one by the front door. Then I went to talk to my neighbor, Lon Miller, about the situation. Lon said he'd do his best to keep an eye out for work that might be being performed when I'm not around.

On August 31, I was at Palomar getting ready for the fall semester, when I needed to call our daughter Darby in Irvine for some reason. In doing so, I used my Sprint Fonecard, like I always do. When I punched in my long distance code information I was told it is invalid. After three failures I called Sprint Customer Relations to find out what the problem was. I was informed, after a lengthy conversation, which included a Pacific Bell representative, that my Sprint service had been canceled on August 25 and another long distance courier subscribed to. Sara had done it of course. All I could think of was that it probably was the result of a cold call. My No Soliciting signs wouldn't work with telephone sales persons. Another problem I hadn't thought of. Anyway I got it changed back to Sprint, who said they would pay for charges to do so. It didn't alleviate the problem I saw ahead though, Sara was easy prey for solicitors over the telephone.

That evening I asked Sara about canceling Sprint. She genuinely acted like she didn't know what I was talking about. She probably didn't either. I knew I had to talk it over with Dr. Smith.

September 9, Sara and I met with Dr. Smith. I informed him of the tree cutting incident, the long distance phone carrier problem and putting up No Solicitation signs. He said, "I'm a doctor, not a lawyer. I have no solution to the problem of Sara making decisions that could affect you financially." He decided to keep Sara's medication on one Haloperidol each day, in the evening, to handle the sun downing effect.

I didn't know a lawyer that dealt with a situation like ours, so I didn't do anything at this time. I did, however, install two smoke alarms in the kitchen area. Sara had burned up two cooking pots in the last month.

Chapter 11

Why Don't You Just Get Out?

*S*ara is starting to leave the lights on all the time now, something she would never have done in the past. She gets up at 6:00 a.m. every morning, even though there is no need to. She cannot make coffee that one can drink, it's so strong it must be diluted. I seem to be doing most of the cooking now, especially on weekends. I don't mind the cooking, it's a good outlet for me. It also seems to take pressure off of Sara, which helps with her moods.

She spends her day playing tennis, coming home, watching the "soaps," and walking down to the mailbox to pick up the mail. Sara's life is void of most of her activities and club gatherings. All that, has disappeared. Her loneliness is increasing although she doesn't outwardly express it lately.

I know I have to do something more for Sara. The way things are going with her, I'm not sure I can finish out this year at Palomar without some kind of help at home. All I can think to do is look into early retirement. I really cannot see trying to teach beyond this year, although I will retire at less than the maximum financial benefit. I would also lose my Palomar medical benefits at age 65. It's apparent though, Sara is beginning to need me fulltime.

I talked to Dr. Smith the third week in September about a new drug called Cognex. Sara's cousin, Doug Stennett the professor in the pharmacy department at OSU, had called me and told me about it. Doug said, "It's designed to impede the progress of Alzheimer's but does not cure it." Dr. Smith said, "I've heard of it, but I'm not familiar with its status. Why don't you call Dr. Brown? He might have more up to date information." I called Dr. Brown, the neurologist, and he said he was aware of it and expected to be educated on its use in the near future. He would let me know then. No doctor would come out and use the word Alzheimer's, only the formal medical term "senile dementia." They all talked around it, and in this case, Cognex specifically says it's to impede the progress of Alzheimer's.

We had another appointment with Dr. Smith for a medication check on Sara. He wanted Sara to take her medication in the evenings. I told him that she would only take it in the morning and I couldn't get her to change. He said if it was too difficult to get her to change, let it go.

Dr. Smith brought up the tree trimming incident. He said that in the foreseeable future, I was going to need to accomplish legal tasks to protect myself financially. He told me he worked with a woman lawyer in San Diego, Mrs. Killen, who was quite familiar with the kind of problems I was having. He assured me that she could help me make some financial decisions and arrangements that would protect me.

All this was certainly new to me, even though I was aware we needed help, it seemed so overwhelming. I knew I should begin to look into it, so I took the number to call.

When I called and made an appointment with the lawyer, I was informed of the cost. Of course, there was no insurance to pay for anything like this, and the cost was high. I agreed. I couldn't think of any other alternative and our doctor had recommended her. I found my way down to San Diego and into some rather fancy law offices like in the movies. No wonder the fees were exorbitant. The lawyer and I discussed the situation and what needed to be done so that the power for decision making and financial affairs could be turned over to me and later to our children. I was a little hesitant, but Mrs. Killen seemed to know what she was talking about and the law firm appeared to have been around for a long time, so I gave the go ahead to do the necessary paperwork.

November 11, Sara and I visited with Dr. Brown to discuss Cognex. One of the first things he asked was if Sara was still driving. I said yes, she had gone to the DMV and taken a driving test. I told him that they did not give her a written examination. He said he was concerned that she had not taken a written exam and I replied that we just did what we were told to do at the DMV. I had the impression he might follow up on his concern about Sara's driving with the DMV. I would just wait and see.

I sent Dr. Brown a copy of a letter I received from Sara's cousin, Doug Stennett, in which he stated his concerns about the drug Cognex. Supposedly the FDA had given an early okay before it was fully tested due to pressure from caregivers. Dr. Brown said that he had read the letter as it pertained to Cognex and indicated that he understood Sara's cousin's concern, but felt responsible to try new things as they became available in order to assist his patients. I asked him if he had ever prescribed the use of Cognex on any other patient and he said that Sara would be the first patient that he was prescribing the drug for, but he was going to start using it with other patients as well.

He gave us an informational kit on Cognex and Alzheimer's. This was the first time that Alzheimer's was actually, fully, being voiced with regard to Sara.

He wrote a prescription for Cognex and said that she was to have her blood tested for a base liver function, which apparently is one of the side affects of the medication.

Dr. Brown asked Sara if she was still volunteering at the hospital. Sara smiled, and said, "Yes." I said nothing, but my body language was apparent that what Sara was saying might be questionable. She had not been to the hospital in months and I believe Dr. Brown knew it.

On the way home Sara was totally confused about what we were doing. I tried to explain to her that we were trying to make things better for her with a new medication. I wanted to read over the material Dr. Brown had given us before I filled the prescription. I also wanted to talk to her cousin Doug about it. I needed to find out what pharmacies carried Cognex and how much it cost. I couldn't get Sara to understand and I was visibly upset.

The next morning I asked Sara to read the information kit about Cognex while I shaved. I knew down deep that reading it would be meaningless to her, but I had to give it a try. About ten minutes later I went into the kitchen and Sara was gone. The information kit on Cognex was in my briefcase. I looked for Sara, but she was gone and so was her car. A few minutes later she returned. I asked where she went and she told me she went to the store to buy some ice cream, but it started to rain, so she came home.

I asked her if she read the information on Cognex. She said, yes. There was no way she could have read it in that amount of time. Then she asked me, "Do you think I have Alzheimer's?" All I could say, sadly, was, "Yes, it's possible." As I recall, that is the first time she actually asked me the question. I told her that the doctors and I are doing all we can to take care of her and help her, regardless of what the problem is. She didn't ask anything else, but just looked despondent.

I went upstairs to do a couple of things and I heard Sara drive off. I have no idea where she was going.

> I'm really getting scared of what is happening, I have absolutely no control of the situation. I keep trying to prevent or avoid problems, but it doesn't seem to work often enough. I am always reacting to problems after they occur.

Over the past months Sara has been functioning less and less as her normal self. She wears the same clothes every day, even the same tennis clothes although she has many to choose from.

She seldom cooks and I have to plan meals for both of us. One day I pulled a chicken out of the freezer to thaw and barbecue. We discussed my plan to barbecue the chicken for dinner a couple of times during the day. I finished working in the garden and came in to start the barbecue. What do you think I found? Sara was frying the chicken as if we had never had any conversation about it.

I called Dr. Brown November 18 and told him I was starting Sara on Cognex. I got Sara's prescription for Haloperidol refilled and had the druggist put directions on the bottle that she was to take it at bedtime.

December 2 was a busy day. We started with a visit to Dr. Smith for a medication check. Then we went to the lab and had Sara provide a blood sample for Dr. Brown to monitor her liver function with while taking Cognex. This blood work has to be done every two weeks while on the Cognex program.

We went home to meet our daughter Darby and then headed to San Diego to meet with the lawyer, Mrs. Killen. We were ushered into a conference room, when we arrived, where the lawyer had all the papers assembled for signature. Darby came with us to witness the proceedings and help her understand what I was doing. The lawyer had prepared six documents for us to sign, which she said would take care of all my concerns.

First there was a Declaration of Trust for the Ellison Family Trust. This document created a living trust, of which I was the trustee and Darby and Corbin would be alternate trustees. Sara was not named a beneficiary of the trust.

All of our assets would need to be moved into this trust instead of being in our names.

Next came the new wills for both of us. They were basically updates of the wills we had prepared previously at the Marine Corps Base, Camp Pendleton legal offices.

A Community Property Agreement and Agreement to Sever Joint Tendencies were next. Everything we owned was in both of our names and this document severed our joint ownership, which would then enable me to act independently as I moved our assets into the trust.

A Quitclaim Deed for personal residence put our house in the family trust. Our house, of course, was our major asset and needed protecting.

Finally a Durable Power of Attorney and Nomination of Conservator was executed. The Durable Power of Attorney gave me full power over Sara's financial and medical matters, including if necessary at a later time to place her in a nursing home. The document also nominated me as the conservator in case Sara became incompetent.

Sara just sat and listened. She didn't ask any questions. We both signed all the documents. Then I gathered the documents and we headed home. Sara usually says nothing during a meeting, but as soon as we leave she has me explain everything to her many times. This time Sara said nothing. She was just quiet.

When we reached home, Sara and Darby went Christmas shopping. I immediately went out and had copies of all the documents made and put the originals in our safety deposit box. I must say I felt some relief. The problem of how to deal with all of this had weighed heavily on me for some time. I don't know how much longer Sara would be considered competent to sign legal papers.

By the end of the day I was very tired, exhausted would be more like it. Next I had to work on moving all of our assets such as our stocks and IRA's into the trust. There wasn't much to move so it didn't take a lot of time.

The next day Darby left me a note when she went home thanking me for trying to help Sara and letting me know that if I needed her she would be just up the road.

On December 4, we were supposed to attend the annual Children's Home Society Christmas Fundraiser. We had gone to this event for years and I usually helped with the parking. Sara purchased tickets for it, but at the last minute decided she did not want to go. I didn't press the issue.

After several days of relative peace, Sara had another bad day. I guess I have never learned what not to say. Why I keep trying to be logical is beyond me. Sara had gone to the store to buy some lettuce and bananas. In less than five minutes after returning home she said, "I'm going back to the store to refill a jug of water." We had eight full jugs on hand. I stupidly said, "Why not do it another time? We have plenty of water. Besides it costs more in gas to get 25 cents in water." She walked across the kitchen and in a very loud voice said, "I am going to get the water!" I have no idea why I said again, "You really don't have to get the water now." At this point Sara yelled, "You son of a bitch. I'm going to do what I want to do!" She came across the room and kicked me saying, "Why don't you just get out?" She hasn't acted like this in some time. I thought the Haloperidol and Cognex were finally really working. She took off, got the water and returned.

December 9 was Sara's 58th birthday. She got up as usual about 6:00 a.m. When Corbin and I got up we found that she had opened all of her cards and presents. She didn't say a word about it being her birthday. For the first time that I can remember, Sara did not bake a birthday cake so I bought one.

A couple of days later I started putting up the Christmas tree. Sara said it was too early, but I finally convinced her it was okay. It was like last year, when she didn't want to put the tree up until the last minute. This was a woman who when Thanksgiving was over would start decorating for Christmas. Not anymore. I had to keep encouraging her to do some decorating around the house. She finally got into the swing of things and seemed to enjoy it.

All summer Sara swam in the pool every day. It wasn't really swimming, she would take a paddleboard and kick back and forth in the pool. She said it helped her back and she no longer was seeing Dr. Bendher. Now the problem was it was late in the year and the water was cold, very cold, but Sara kept going into the pool. No matter how hard I tried, I could not get her to stop going in. I finally called Dr. Smith and told him my problem. He called Sara and told her to stop going into the pool. She finally stopped.

Just before Christmas I decided it was time to fully explain to our friends and family what Sara was going through. Some of them knew a little and some knew nothing, but rather than let rumors fill the vacuum, I decided to fill it with the truth. Sara had been so personable throughout the years and had kept up with everyone. I sent a blanket letter to Sara's friends and relatives explaining the best I could what was happening. I used the word Alzheimer's now. I would end up doing this every year at Christmas. I suggested that if anyone would like to talk to Sara they do it now, because I was not sure what the future would be like.

Sara got a call from her mother the day before Christmas. Sara's only uncle by marriage had died. Sara seemed saddened by the news, but otherwise didn't seem upset at all. Sara seemed to have lost all emotion, except when she was angry.

I got to celebrate today by installing a new disposal for the kitchen sink. Sara sat and stared at me. I tried to engage her by asking for some help with a couple of things, but that didn't work. She didn't have much spark.

Darby, Corbin and Amy all made it home for Christmas. Darby and Amy brought their dogs. Sara seemed to enjoy the dogs and of course our own Spud got into the swing of things.

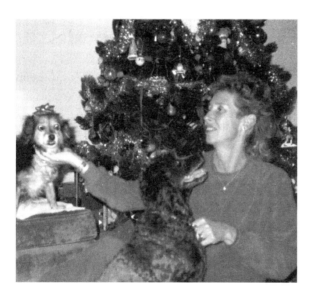

Christmas morning came, but it just lacked the spirit it used to hold. I got Sara a new tennis outfit and a case of tennis balls. Sara actually showed a little enthusiasm over her gifts.

Brother Don dropped by to say hello and enjoyed playing with all the dogs. He left Pat at home cooking the turkey. We had our dinner and one of Corbin's friends from the Marine Corps joined us.

December 27 is my 59th birthday. Everyone was leaving early, so we celebrated a day early. I didn't get much, but then I didn't ask for anything. However this is the first time Sara has not given me a gift and a card, it didn't even seem to register with her that it was my birthday.

After everyone left, I took Sara to the movies to see *Tombstone.* As always she just sat there and never made a sound. When we got home Sara wanted to take down all the Christmas decorations. I wasn't going to argue, so we had everything down and put away in about an hour. It seemed to satisfy her.

Sara ended the year on December 31 by going to see Dr. Bendher, which was a surprise. I remembered Dr. Bendher calling me about Sara being upset with her and her staff. Sara might not remember, though, I'm not sure. I guess everything went well because I didn't hear from the doctor. Maybe Sara's medication is working after all. Her emotional flare ups are less often now.

Chapter 12

What's True?
What's Fantasy?

ara started the New Year off playing tennis. Her usual time to play was 9:00 a.m., but she came home early, by 9:30 a.m. She said, "Everyone just left early." I note that most times now when she comes home from tennis, regardless of the time, she says, "Everyone left early."

We watched the Rose Bowl football game together New Year's afternoon. I thought back to our college days when, on New Year's Day in 1957, I played both offensive and defensive guard in the Rose Bowl against the University of Iowa on my college football team, Oregon State. I remembered that Sara came to Pasadena with her father for the game. Sara never lost the enthusiastic personality she acquired during three years as a cheerleader in high school. Although I couldn't see her from the field, I knew she had been cheering our team.

After the game, I went out to the barn to feed Spot, the cat. I saw Sara come out of the house and start walking up the road. I asked her where she was going and she replied, "To check the mail."

I reminded her that today was a holiday and there was no mail. She turned around and went back to the house. I then heard the front door being slammed as hard as possible several times. I hurried back to the house and found Sara in the kitchen. I asked her what was wrong and she went crazy! She had the dinner napkins and rings in her hand, turned and threw them at the kitchen cabinets. She turned and started to hit and kick me. She screamed, "I want out of here!" Then she told me, "Just kill me!" and "I want a divorce!" I was scared, but didn't try to restrain her, as I felt that would have made it even worse.

Her fury didn't last long though. After a minute or so she quieted down and went about doing things in the kitchen. I guess telling her it was a holiday just set her off. Or maybe it was my tone of voice, I'm not really sure. There's no way to tell anymore what will cause her emotions to erupt.

Sara's outburst in the kitchen solves one mystery for me. I have noticed some dents in the cabinets, windowsills and frames, now I have an idea what has been happening. I remembered one time as I drove in the driveway, I saw her slamming a metal dustpan to the surface of the driveway so hard she bent it out of shape. At the time it looked like she was trying to hit our dog Spud. I felt so bad when I saw this. Sara really needed Spud, and I felt responsible for Spud's safety also. What a dilemma!

On Monday, I called Dr. Smith and left a message regarding Sara's recent outbreak. He returned the call and left a message, saying, "Increase Sara's medication." His message sounded so simple, but to myself I said, "Right, and how am I going to increase her medication without upsetting her and throwing her into confusion?" I couldn't figure out how to follow his instructions so I decided the safest and best way to get her medication increased was for Dr. Smith to tell her. The constant figuring out of how to be helpful, and not hurtful or controlling, was taking its toll on me.

On January 5, I got a call from Amy who was quite upset. She asked me, "Did you know that mother sent me a package?" I said, "I don't know of any package." Amy told me, "While I was there over Christmas, I brought some frozen diet food with me. I forgot to take some of it home with me and left it there in the freezer."

Apparently when Sara found it, she packaged up the frozen food and mailed it to Amy. Amy was shocked. She said, "I can't believe Mom mailed me frozen food." I was sad for Amy. I hoped the kids could be spared some of the craziness, but they are getting involved more and more.

A couple of days later I was pruning some trees. Sara came outside and started pacing back and forth in the driveway. It was the first time I noticed her pacing. She said nothing, but just paced slowly back and forth.

Then on January 10, I came home around noon and Sara was gone. I looked at her calendar and it had "Lab Test," written down. I called the lab where Sara had her blood work done. They said she had just left. What? That can't be! Sara is supposed to have her blood work done every two weeks. We just had it done last week. I know, I'm the one who takes her for the testing. Why would she go on her own, a week early? It doesn't make sense. I couldn't see what saying anything to her about it would accomplish though, so when she returned home I just let it go.

A few days went by and I took Sara to our bank to have some stock certificates endorsed for placement into the family trust. I thought there might be a problem, but there wasn't. It all went well. Sara talked to one of the employees at the bank, Ruth, a friend she had known for years. When we were leaving, Ruth said, "Sara didn't seem to be her usual 'sparky' self." Another friend who doesn't yet know.

I came home around noon on January 19. I noted that Sara was to go to a Panhellenic luncheon, I'm not sure why. I thought she had dropped her participation. She came home around 1:30 p.m. and I asked her how the luncheon went. In a frustrated tone of voice she said, "I didn't go. I couldn't find the place." I could only imagine how frustrated Sara must be when she couldn't find places she had known before. I just wish I had the time to take her everywhere she needed to go.

> She hasn't washed any clothes, towels or bedding in some time. It's to the point I realize that I'll need to start doing the washing myself. I

encourage her to do some things and she says yes at the time, but then nothing happens. I don't dare make an issue out of it. Instead I keep trying to remember the medical reports, especially "nothing can be done." The decline will continue and there is no turning back. The medication is only going to delay the deterioration, not turn it around. It's strictly a coping measure, not a cure.

We visit Dr. Smith on January 20 and he increases Sara's medication slightly. He also tells us that I am to give Sara additional medication as required for episodes of hostility. I keep trying to remember, hostility is normal, not abnormal for someone in Sara's condition.

I left my car at a local service station for some work on my windshield wipers. I asked Sara the night before, "Would you drop me off to pick up my car on your way to play tennis?" She nodded yes. In the morning she was not dressed for tennis when it was time to go. I reminded her to get changed so she could play tennis and on the way drop me off at the service station. While she went in to change into her tennis clothes, I went outside to wait. She came out soon, got into the car and backed out. But she turned the wheels too far. Her front bumper caught on the garage door springs and door frame, which almost ripped the bumper off. You would have thought she would get out to look. No! You would have thought this would have upset her. No! It's as if it didn't even happen.

One day I bought a can of stewed tomatoes for dinner. I placed the can on the kitchen counter and told Sara, "We can have them along with dinner." Then I went out and worked in the garden for awhile. When I came back in, the can of tomatoes was no longer on the kitchen counter. Sara was cooking peas. I just thought she wanted peas, which was fine with me, so I didn't say anything.

The next day when I was fixing lunch and went to the pantry for something. I saw the can of tomatoes with dents in it. It looked as if it had been thrown several times very hard on the floor. I took the can out to Sara and asked, "What happened?" She looked at it and said timidly, "It was the earthquake." Her answer was almost funny, I had to smile. A few days earlier we had a little earthquake, but it hardly rattled the windows. Plus. . .I bought the tomatoes after the earthquake. It is becoming more apparent that Sara has spells of anger and confusion even when I am not around to take the brunt of it. I'm becoming worried that Sara might hurt herself in one of her rages.

Corbin came home on January 22. It was good for me to be able to talk to Corbin about his mother even though there was nothing either of us could do. I told him about Sara getting lost looking for her luncheon and about the tomato can incident. Corb rarely says anything when I talk to him about Sara's condition, but then what is there to say. He does listen though, which is helpful. As I talked to Corb, I realized I was feeling scared, almost to the point of being nonfunctional myself.

I have so many things to do in preparation for the start of spring semester at Palomar, but I can't seem to concentrate on getting them done, which is totally unlike me. With school starting Monday and having to leave Sara home alone so much, I'm really worried. For sure, I must make some serious plans about retiring at the end of the semester even though it will seriously affect our income.

Took Sara for her blood test on January 27. Thus far there has been no noticeable impact on Sara's liver functioning as it pertains to her taking Cognex. That's some good news!

I had to go to a CCA meeting in San Francisco this weekend, but I decided I could no longer go off and leave Sara alone for a weekend. I would now have to start depending on the kids to help, which I didn't like, even though it was necessary. Amy agreed to come down from Long Beach and stay with Sara while I was gone. I planned to ask, whichever of our children are available, for help each time I had to go away.

Needless to say, I was reading up on Alzheimer's. In hindsight, I would have to say Sara's fraternal grandmother had Alzheimer's. She was in her eighties when she could no longer recognize anyone and was put in a nursing home. I learned that's the age, about eighty-five, when one out of three contract the disease. Sara has what is called early-onset Alzheimer's and it is much more rare, although there have been cases reported of people contracting it in their twenties.

I found that Alzheimer's is a long, debilitating disease that destroys the brain over a ten to twenty year period. When I tried to find the answer about how long I could expect Sara to live, I found Alzheimer's would cut Sara's life expectancy by about one third. That meant we would have to deal with this for many years to come. I needed to brace myself for the years ahead.

As I looked for a reason why Sara contracted the disease so early, it was speculation. Sara's mother often blamed herself for Sara's condition, remembering all too well Sara's birth in which she didn't let out a sound for four grueling hours. Sara was a "blue baby" which is a name given to babies born to parents of incompatible blood types.

Another theory is that a virus that lay dormant in the body for some time could cause Alzheimer's. I remember in the early eighties, Sara had a bad case of Hepatitis B, which was discovered when she was giving blood. Her skin turned yellow and she was low on energy for some time.

Sara had upper respiratory infections also, which I believe began when she nearly died of pneumonia at around a year old. What concerned me more though, was how to deal with Alzheimer's. Whatever the cause, it was now a fact that we had to deal with today.

I found a national association had been formed called the Alzheimer's Association. Naturally, I sent away for everything I could find, as well as reading several books on the subject. I began to look through the services and support groups to see if I could find some help.

I discovered that the disease impairs many cognitive functions besides memory. Abstract thought declines, as well as the ability to carry out complex thought processes. Also, much to my surprise, I discovered symptoms might appear twenty to forty years before they are diagnosed.

I must say, in looking back over our time together, which is almost forty years, I'm not sure that Sara was ever really good at abstract thinking or grasping complex issues. As I think back on it, I remember her father cautioning me that Sara needed to be taken care of.

When interviewed, our eldest daughter Darby recounted what seems to me to be quite accurate, that reasoning was not how Sara dealt with life. Sara had a set of rules: what was wrong, what was right, what was good, what's bad, what to do and what not to do. For example: French kissing was yucky; you never divorced; you didn't get a bicycle until you were ten, and girls don't call boys. The list was endless, but it gave Sara security in knowing the right thing to do in most of life's circumstances.

As I understood more about the disease, I began to look through the services and support groups to see if I could find some help. I found that there are daycare services for Alzheimer's victims, as well as persons with other types of mental problems.

As I read through the symptoms and stages, I discovered there are three predominant states that occur before the final state. The first stage lasts about two years: The afflicted individual has an inability to deal with numbers or finances, has difficulty recalling certain words and names of friends, can't keep track of where they left things, such as keys, and they get lost traveling to familiar places. They are unable to recall what happened just a few minutes ago or to remember what they read in the paper or hear on television or radio about current events. They have difficulty counting backward by fours or sevens. They also have a decrease in emotional response, which is called a "flattening effect."

The second stage, which is called moderate stage, can last two to ten years: They are not able to remember simple details of their life such as where they live, their phone number, the phone numbers of friends and family. No longer do they measure their life by time, whether it is the hour, day, season or year—they live in an "eternal present."

Deciding what to wear becomes a huge, complex problem, so they pick the old, more familiar, not the new, which is confusing. At this stage, there is no separation of time between now and the past. What happened twenty years ago may seem like now, or yesterday. Everything is now, there is no past, and all events in their life are meshed together, not separated. They forget the schools they attended or they remember the past as now. At this stage, anyone who knew them earlier in their lives will indeed recognize that something is deeply wrong with the person.

Third Stage: They alienate the very family members and caregivers upon whom they have become dependant. They may exhibit bizarre behavior, become angry and irrational and want to kill themselves. They become paranoid and have delusional thinking. Their vocabulary diminishes drastically and their motor skills diminish as the part of the brain that governs the physical body crashes, resulting in urinary and bowel incontinence. Unfortunately, this stage can last up to seven years. Along the way the vocabulary dwindles to about a dozen words, and then to just one or two words—yes or no. By now, the person loses the ability to walk, to hold their head upright and begins to disappear into a vegetative state, losing all control over the body.

The very final stage is regression to the level of a newborn: Not being able to hold up their head or even smile, and then finally, lapsing into a coma.

Very few Alzheimer's victims ever get to these last stages, as they contract other illnesses that bring on their death, usually pneumonia or infections due to their incontinence, malnutrition, dehydration or heart disease. As Sara contracted the illness so early in her life and had been so physically active playing tennis daily, I could only surmise that we would go through all the stages before her spirit would be freed from her body.

It was easy to pick out the steps we had already taken, although I found some of the stages overlap each other. The information I was gaining gave me understanding of the steps ahead in a long, long journey, one in which Sara would unquestionably disappear from my life into a world only she knew.

On February 2, I decided to visit a daycare center in Oceanside. Maybe it might be a solution to Sara staying home all alone. I met with one of the social workers, Bob Triple. I discussed our situation with Bob and he did not paint a very pretty picture. He remarked, "Some caregivers just abandon their problem person." He pointed to a woman and said, "Her husband just up and left her." I recalled reading about an Alzheimer's victim who was found abandoned sitting in a wheelchair at a racetrack somewhere.

Anyway, this daycare center provided a five day a week care service for mentally impaired persons, at a cost. I already checked and knew that I had no insurance that would pay for any kind of daycare services. Still, I filled out the necessary papers. He said, "We'll keep them on file for an indefinite period of time and I'll call you at such time we might decide to update our files and throw away old data."

The next day we met with Dr. Brown. Both of us agreed that the 10mg dosage of Cognex was not providing any sign of results for Sara, so he was increasing the dosage to 20mg. We were to meet in six weeks for another evaluation.

I decided it was time to rotate our bed mattress, and it would be an incentive to change the bed sheets, which had not been done in some time. After stripping the bed and turning the mattress, Sara started remaking the bed using the same sheets. I suggested that we put on some clean new sheets. Fortunately she did not have a problem with that, and we made the bed together.

I got her to wash the sheets and also the clothes she had been wearing for the last couple of weeks. However, after she washed and dried her clothes, she changed right back into them. Guess it is to be her regular uniform, worn each day. She has closets full of clothes, in our room, upstairs and in the girl's rooms. She could wear a different outfit everyday and it would take a year to wear them all at least once.

One day I brought home some chicken fajitas and tortillas for dinner. Sara liked this dinner. She got out what we called her "salad shooter." It cuts up cheese and all kinds of stuff, but she was cutting the cheese by hand. I asked her if she could fix some lettuce for the fajitas. She tried to put some lettuce through the "salad shooter," but couldn't figure out how to work it. I never did know how to work it. She couldn't get it to work, so she just said, "I don't want any lettuce." I went back to the cutting board to cut some lettuce because I did want some lettuce, and I knew that Sara did too. I feel so sad for Sara, things that used to be so routine and so simple are now monumental tasks, and some are no longer possible.

I visited another adult daycare center facility on February 7. It was similar to the first one, but the hours were not as good, although it was closer to home. Anyway I took notes of my observations and put them into my ever growing files.

It was about time to take the plunge and see if I could find some support for myself. I attended an Alzheimer's support group meeting. I have never been much of one for group therapy, but I did see what I was going through now was nothing like it could be in the future.

One woman said she had been a caregiver for twelve years, first for her mother and now for her husband. She said one thing I could see would be a problem, and that was when they have to give up driving. Everyone at the meeting had a little different story to tell. I noticed I was the only male present. The women told stories about dealing with their husbands. They all seemed to make so light of their situation.

On February 11, I took Sara to see Dr. Jones. Sara must be tested for TB if she is ever going to participate in daycare, so I thought I might as well have it done. Dr. Jones had not seen Sara in quite some time. He asked her, "Do you still volunteer at our local hospital?" Sara smiled and said, "Yes, I do." She has not been there for over a year now.

I had a CCA meeting this weekend in San Francisco and Amy came home to stay with Sara. I called home Friday night and asked Sara, "How did your dentist appointment go today?" Sara answered, "Just fine." I talked to Amy and Amy said, "I called ahead about Mom's appointment just to double check. The receptionist said Mom had no appointment." Guess we are learning that what Sara says, is not necessarily factual and, to make sure, you have to double check. When I got home, Amy had nothing negative to report, she just said, "All went well." I loaded Amy down with oranges and vegetables from the garden. As she prepared to leave, Amy said, "My two dogs really like to visit because they get to run around the backyard."

For the first time, this Valentine's Day, Sara had nothing for me. I remembered it had been Sara who taught me early in our marriage about birthdays, holidays and special occasions. I even found out when my mother and father's birthdays were. Birthdays had never been an event in my family and not much attention had been paid to special occasions. Sara was always on top of these things and made sure cards were sent and presents given. Now all that seems to be part of her past. I'm the one remembering now. I got Sara a card that said, 'You're My Sweetheart' and a box of candy to go with the card. She looked at the card, but never read it. When I came home after work though, she had a very nice card for me. I guess she went out and got it while I was at work.

My usual poker parlor was having an Omaha poker tournament, which was one of my favorite poker games, on Sunday the 20th of February. It was raining and there wasn't much I could do outside, so I vacuumed the house and dusted. After lunch Sara was engrossed in TV and I went to play in the tournament, and won! What a nice payoff! Now that's my kind of therapy!

Chapter 13

What Was That
Check For?

$\mathcal{J}$ decided I would take Sara out for Chinese food and celebrate my tournament win, rather than stop, shop, go home and cook dinner. I called, but there was no answer. I called again, again and again, but no answer. I hurried home. She was there, so I asked her, "Why didn't you answer the phone?" She said, "I did, but no one was there." I knew I had called over six times and let it ring and ring. She just never answered. I didn't understand . . . did she really think she answered it?

Corbin came home one Saturday to help me transport an aerator for the lawn. I was wearing some new overalls I had bought and cut off the trouser legs because they were too long. Sara said, "I would like to put a hem in them." I said, "Okay." She had tried before, but gave up because she couldn't figure out how to get the sewing machine to work. Sure enough, she came back from her sewing machine saying, "The sewing machine didn't work." Sewing had been one of Sara's favorite past times. She used to sew clothes for the kids, dresses for herself and shirts for me.

Then on the 1st of March, I would have to say I saw remarkable improvement in Sara. Possibly the Cognex was having a favorable affect. She picked flowers for the house, swept the patio and walkways, washed clothes, washed her hair, changed clothes two days in a row, fed Spot and picked up oranges that had fallen off the trees. She has done all of this on her own with not a word from me. This is a decided change in her behavior! It didn't last long though—in the same week, I came home one night to find the furnace going full blast, with the heat on high. I went into the bedroom and found the sliding door to the pool wide open and cold air roaring in. Sara is continually leaving doors and windows open and lights on. She doesn't even lock up the house any longer. I remember that in the past these were all big issues for her, i.e., lights off, doors closed and locked.

Saturday, March 4, I was scheduled to give a CPR class at Palomar. It was an all day event for which I had put in my support requests some weeks in advance. On Friday, I was checking to make sure everything was ready to go. Nothing was! I found failure at every turn. It was hard to cope with failure at work and at home.

I finally got home looking for peace and quiet. I found a message on our answering service saying, "Mrs. Ellison, please call [our bank] about your account." I decided to return the call. Sara was overdrawn by $330 in her checking account. I ask Sara, "Can I see your checkbook?" It showed a balanced of $18,000! A simple review of the entries showed she had made a $10,000 error in addition. I quickly tried to balance the numbers. The best I could tell there should have been a balance of $660. I told Sara that we would take care of this on Monday. I took her checkbook and put in my briefcase.

In preparation for the next day's all day CPR class, I set up the coffee maker in the kitchen for a big pot of coffee in the morning, and went to bed. I got up at 6:00 a.m., but Sara beat me by a few minutes. I went out to get some breakfast and my coffee for my all day class. I looked at the coffee decanter, it was nearly empty, only a cup or so left. Sara had poured the coffee out down to the usual daily level. She poured at least six cups of coffee down the drain. When I checked my briefcase I noticed her checkbook was gone.

She had taken it back. I had no time to take care of this at the moment. I had to get going to my CPR class.

When I got back from the CPR class around 5:00 p.m., I asked Sara for our joint checking account checkbook. On opening it up I saw a check for "Sara" for $300 written today. I asked, "What was the check for?" She replied, "To cover the shortage in my account. I took care of it today." On further investigation I found out she had not taken care of the shortage, instead she had taken out the $300 in cash. I lost my patience and took the money away from her as well as taking her checkbook again. I said with finality, "We will both go to the bank on Monday and get it straightened out."

> That's enough, I've put it off as long as I can. I am closing her account on Monday, one way or another . . . if necessary by the power of attorney she signed earlier! I am exhausted.

I thought all day Sunday about the situation. I decided to eliminate all of Sara's access to our family finances. The one area I had a problem with was our joint checking account since I receive checks to this account and needed to keep it open. I planned, however, to take over total check writing responsibility. For sure her private account had to go if I wanted to prevent more financial headaches.

On Monday we went to the lab for a blood test, then to see Dr. Smith. Dr. Smith approved of my taking control of all of the family assets to keep Sara from making mistakes. I told him about investigating daycare facilities. He, too, thought it would be a good idea if Sara could participate in some out of home activity.

We left Dr. Smith and headed to Sara's bank to resolve her checking account problem. It turns out she was overdrawn by $345.20. We had talked about closing the account for the past two days, but she kept asking the same question over and over again, "If the account is closed, what will happen to the money?" No matter how many times I explained it to her, she didn't understand that the account was overdrawn and we would have to pay money to close it. It was a concept she couldn't grasp. It was not a fun day. I got the account closed and also got my name added to a savings account Sara had at the bank. She couldn't write checks against it so I didn't see that as a problem.

> Later I will withdraw the proceeds so she cannot have access to them. Not now though, this was enough for both of us. I may have to use the power of attorney if I'm not able to close the savings account without her signature. Will get to that at a later time.

On March 9, I attended another Alzheimer's support group meeting. I remarked to myself, "I can't believe the hell some have been going through." One woman was late due to her husband taking his bowel movement and smearing it on the walls. This wasn't the first time he had done that and she had a time cleaning it up. A common story was the Alzheimer's person running away and getting lost. Another common theme was trying to find ways to keep their partners from escaping.

Apparently I am only at the "tip of the iceberg."

The next day, Sara left for tennis at her usual time. On the way to Palomar I went by the tennis courts to see how she was doing. Everything looked fine and she was enjoying her game. When I got home, Sara said, "We received a bill from Dr. Smith, but it was for too much money. I ripped it up and threw it away." Immediately, I went to search the trash for it. I found the parts and taped them back together. The bill actually showed we owed nothing, but looking in the trash revealed that she had torn up a certificate for shares of common stock that I had just put into the family trust. I retrieved the certificate and taped it together knowing it was going to take some time and effort to get a replacement. At least I thought, "I was fortunate to find it." By this time I was upset and shaking, not just inside, but outside now too.

I went looking for our joint checkbook and found Sara had once again taken it out of my briefcase. Sometimes I just forget to lock it. This is not a fun time! I told Sara, "I need our joint checkbook." I found she had written a check to the lab where she had her blood work done. I asked Sara, "Where is the statement from the lab for your blood work?" Sara said, "I can't find it." I went to the trash, but it's not there either. Once more I took the checkbook and locked it in my briefcase. Now I'd have to remember to keep it locked.

I started thinking about some mail I know I should have received, including occasional bills I can't find. It was time to do something about the mail. The best solution I could think of was to get a post office box. I did that and then sent out a change of address to all important entities, banks, credit cards, and anyone else I considered important. I informed all close relatives of the post office box, "If you want to ensure I get the mail, send your correspondence to the post office box." This left unimportant mail and junk mail to be delivered to our mailbox at home. Sara told me when I asked her about the mail, "People are stealing it." If that were the least bit true, if they stole it now they wouldn't be getting much.

I am to the point I can barely function at Palomar. I am doing a lousy job of teaching and I'm sure my students know it. Once again, I put it in my mind to retire, even though I don't act on it.

March 12, I made a one day trip to San Francisco for a CCA meeting. It's another area that I must admit to myself I'm not doing a very good job at now. Corbin came and stayed with Sara. He took her to a movie.

The return plane flight was delayed for five hours, so I didn't get home until very late. Sara was up, and I asked her, "What movie did you go to? Was it any good?" Sara said, "I don't remember the name or what it was about."

I went to another Alzheimer's support group meeting March 16. I'm not sure where the "support" term comes from? I guess just talking about all the problems caregivers go through and having someone to listen to your story is what it is all about. I hear of no real solutions to problems. Sadly I was beginning to realize that there just might be no solutions, only help in learning to cope with problems that progressively worsen. I found the meetings very depressing.

I took Sara to the lab for her blood work on March 17, and then to see Dr. Brown, the neurologist. He decided to move Sara's

Cognex dosage up from 20mg to 40mg. I told him that I could see no real positive changes in Sara's condition. He said, "I have to admit that Sara is my first patient I have prescribed Cognex for. Like many of my colleagues, this is all new to us. Sara's blood tests are good. After a month on 40mg dosage, I will coordinate with Dr. Smith and Dr. White to have Sara retested for her cognitive skills. That will give me a comparison of eighteen months since Sara was first evaluated by Dr. White."

Dr. Brown again asked, "Is Sara still driving?" I said, "Yes, she has been tested and seems to be driving well." He just shook his head, like he was perplexed.

Its still March, but soon it will be May, that's when Amy is to be married. Plans are moving in that direction, but Sara can't really be of help. Darby came home the weekend of March 19 and took Sara out shopping in preparation for a wedding shower for Amy. Darby said, "While shopping I saw some loose checks in Mom's purse." Darby took Sara to the movies and after they left, I checked Sara's purse. She did have blank checks from our bank. On further investigation I found she had taken three checks I had forgotten about out of my desk drawer. When I think I have everything covered, Sara proves I haven't.

Sara's mother called and asked if I could bring Sara up to see her. So we took a trip to Placerville on March 29 for three days. Sara packed for the trip with a miscellaneous selection of clothes. I had to add some items to make sure she had enough, including a sweater. After two days, I had to "force" her to change her clothes. Since I checked every night, I asked on the second night, "Did you take your medication at bedtime?" Sara smiled and said, "Yes, I did." The next morning I found out she hadn't. It is to the point, there is no way I can believe what Sara tells me. I don't think she really lies, she just doesn't remember. She seems to answer yes to most any question whether her doctors, or I, ask it, she just agrees with anything asked. The way I saw our trip, it wasn't bad, it was actually better than normal. Sara's mother hadn't been around her though, and was shocked. She said, "I just can't believe what is happening to my daughter, I just can't."

Easter Sunday came and all the kids were home. Darby made nice Easter baskets for presents. This is the first year Sara didn't treat it as a special occasion. I got her an Easter lily. Sara was oblivious to the day she used to enjoy so much. I remembered with fondness that Sara used to fix up the eggs for hiding, and I'd hide them. Then the kids would go off for the hunt.

I took Sara to the lab for her blood work on April 7. When we left home she started to cry. I asked her, "What's wrong, Sara?" She just said, "I don't know." After awhile she stopped crying. I didn't know what to say, so I just said nothing but I felt so sorry for her, and maybe for me also.

After the lab visit we had to take Spud to the vet for a rabies shot. Sara had sent in the license fee, but neglected to get the required rabies shot. This is one of the reasons I have to open all of her mail and check the trash to see what she might have thrown away. She still gets mail for things she used to handle routinely, like the dog licenses. Either she doesn't read her mail, or reads it, doesn't understand it and throws it away.

> In the last couple of weeks, Sara continues to do those things she wants or likes to do. She puts out the garbage, picks up fallen oranges, weeds a little, gets her car washed and oil changed. But she's almost totally quit cleaning the house. When she dusts, it is a poor job, and I have to redo it.

On Saturday, April 9, I ask Sara if she'd like to go to the movies, he says yes, but a short time later she says, "I want to have my hair done for Amy's shower tomorrow." I told her that would be fine. Then I call her hairdresser Gladis, and make an appointment for 1:30 p.m.

A short time later Sara asks, "When are we going to the movie?" I said, "We are not going to the movie because you are having your hair done for Amy's shower." A short time later she puts on her coat and hat, because it is raining, and says, "I'm ready for the movie." I tell her again, "You have a hair appointment at 1:30 p.m." Because it is raining and she is so confused, I decided I should take her, instead of letting her drive. I had the check made out to the hairdresser, Gladis. When we got to the beauty parlor, Gladis said, "Sara needs a little more than a wash and blow dry today." I said, "Fine, do what you think she needs."

I had an hour or so to wait, so I went outside. Next door to the beauty parlor was a big room where I have often seen people playing cards, but never knew what it was all about. So, with nothing else to do except wait for Sara, I went in to inquire what was going on. The person in charge said, "This is a duplicate bridge club, where people come in to play bridge on a daily basis." I knew what bridge was and had even tried playing it once or twice while in the Marine Corps, but really didn't know much about it. He showed me around and explained how duplicate bridge was played and how it was scored. It looked very interesting, even to a person who had played poker for years. "Anyway," he said, "we have a beginner's class on Monday afternoons if you are interested." I said, "I am, but right now I don't have time. Possibly some time in the future."

When I picked Sara up, I gave Gladis the check and said, "I must owe you more for the extra work." Gladis said, "No, everything is fine." I could see that Gladis also noticed the dramatic change in Sara.

On Sunday, I took Sara to Amy's shower in Long Beach. We stopped and had lunch before I took her to Amy's apartment. They needed some flowers, so I left Sara and went to buy some flowers. When I came back with the flowers, I left Sara with Darby and Amy at about 12:45 p.m. and went to find a nearby park with a place to sit to work on a lecture for my first aid class. I called Amy at around 3:00 p.m. and asked, "How are things going?" Amy replied, "Mom is ready to leave and she said she didn't think you were coming back after her." I rushed back to Amy's, and as I walked in, Sara grabbed her purse and started out the door. I had to ask her to please wait a minute so I could say goodbye to everyone. Amy said the shower went fine and that Sara did okay. I took pictures when we first got there, and later I noticed how beautiful Sara looked in them. The pictures just don't show what is happening to her.

Our 32nd wedding anniversary is April 14. I got her a card. She got me a card also, but hers was from a "third person." It was like it was from someone else, but it was signed, "I Love You, Sara."

I had already asked Sara, "What would you like for our anniversary?" She said with a smile, "Just you."

It's times like this that make this nightmare somewhat bearable.

Chapter 14

I'll Drive You

On April 21, I came home to pick Sara up for a lab visit, but she wasn't home. I waited until about 2:00 p.m. when she showed up. I inquired, "Where have you been?" She replied, "I went to the Boy's and Girl's Club fashion show luncheon. I was supposed to meet two friends there, but they didn't show up. I stayed anyway and sat with some people I didn't know. We had a salad and strawberries for lunch and I had a good time." It was almost like the Sara of old, having a good time with people.

On Friday, April 22, I had to go to a CCA meeting in San Francisco. Amy came down from Long Beach to stay with Sara. My flight back Saturday night was delayed an hour. This was the fourth trip in a row the return flight has been delayed. I had decided over the weekend that I was in fact going to retire from Palomar. This time I didn't just keep it to myself, I even told Amy of my decision. Monday I planned to start the formal paper work to get it done.

A week later, I met with Dr. Smith in his San Diego office. I told him Sara had been shaking and crying for the past few days. He thought about it and called the poison control center. He asked, "Is there any possible interaction between Haloperidol and Cognex?" The response on the other end of the telephone was, "No."

I talked to him about entering Sara into an Alzheimer's research project for a new medication. He said he did not think Sara was a good candidate for such a research study, because it would require she be taken off of Haloperidol. He didn't think it was worth the risk with her history of past violence. I understood his viewpoint, but was somewhat disappointed. I guess it's hard to give up hope entirely, and there are constantly new research projects springing up as scientists are trying to find new remedies for the disease. I'm just hoping that because Sara is so young, indeed there will be a miracle drug discovered before she becomes really elderly.

May 1, my last month at Palomar starts. This past week I have observed Sara withdraw more and more. She appears to not be playing tennis, at least the last three days. She doesn't talk unless asked a specific question and the response is "yes" or "no." She is too quiet. She just sits and watches TV. I don't think she is feeding Spud everyday, because Spud is always scratching at her dog dish, at which time I feed her. Sara seems to be getting no benefit from Cognex.

I mailed my retirement papers to the State Teachers Retirement System in Sacramento May 1. I plan to retire on May 27.

May 1 also marked my official retirement from real estate. My job will soon be that of fulltime caregiver.

On May 3, Sara got up at 1:30 a.m. and went into the bathroom. I asked, "What are you doing up at this hour?" Sara answered, "I'm getting some Tum's for my stomach." She then left the bathroom, and bedroom. After a few minutes she was not back, so I got up to check on her. I found her in the living room lying on the sofa. I asked her "What are you doing in here?" She replied, "Sleeping." I said, "Please come back to bed." She did.

On arising in the morning, I asked her, "Are you going to play tennis this morning?" She nodded her head and replied, "No." I noted she had not played tennis since the last Thursday, so I inquired further, "Why aren't you going to play?" Sara didn't answer—she was silent. Then she walked away as if I wasn't even there waiting for an answer.

On May 5, we met with Dr. Smith, the psychiatrist. He had talked to Dr. Brown, the neurologist, and they agreed that Dr. White, the psychologist, should retest Sara, since it had been over a year. Dr. Brown did not feel the Cognex was having any positive results, but he wanted to have Sara tested while she was still on it.

Dr. Smith asked Sara, "What have you been doing today?" She replied, "Watching TV." Then he asked her, "Which show did you watch? Who was in it?" Sara replied, "I don't really know. I just enjoyed watching." I volunteered, "We go to the movies often, but Sara doesn't remember the movie we see. Later when I try to discuss the movie with her, she doesn't remember what it was about. She also doesn't express any reaction while watching. She makes no sounds at all." Then I realized, as I was speaking to Dr. Smith, "You know, Sara never laughs anymore, but she still continues her wonderful smile."

A couple of days later, after much coaxing, I got Sara to wash her clothes. Then I got her to wash her hair, which was greatly needed. I checked on her as she was washing her hair and saw she was just washing the top of her head, so I helped her get the sides and back. Next I'd have to try to get her to take a bath.

Mother's Day was May 8. Sara got up early to go to the bathroom. When I got up, I noted she had messed all over the toilet seat and had made a poor effort to clean it off. I gave her a card and a new night gown and robe. She showed no interest, never opening the envelope to read the card or take the gown and robe out of the box. No reaction whatsoever.

I had to go San Francisco on May 13 to a CCA State Council meeting for three days. Darby came down to stay with Sara. When I got home, Darby said, "I got Mom to take a bath, but I couldn't get her to wash her hair. Otherwise, everything went well." I appreciated that Darby had done a lot of cleaning.

On Monday, Sara got a phone call. I happened to overhear Sara talking to a woman about tennis. The woman wanted to play with Sara on Wednesday to which Sara agreed to, and then she hung up the phone. Sara said, irately, "I will not play tennis with 'that woman'." She had just agreed to play, and then, within seconds, said she would not. I asked her who the woman was so I could call the woman back. Sara just said, "I don't remember her name."

In preparation for retirement, the Palomar College Faculty Association of the CTA/CCA/NEA gave a retirement party for four of us that were retiring. I had been a member since 1982 and had served as secretary for several years and finally as vice-president. Sara attended with me and surprisingly had a really good time. I was glad, Sara certainly deserved having a good time. She had been such a supportive and active worker in our collective bargaining efforts just a few years earlier.

Amy and Marc's wedding was set for Saturday, May 21. Friday I packed us up, trying not to leave anything important behind. We got to Long Beach and checked into our motel. Then we went to the wedding rehearsal and all went well.

At age 24, Amy was married in a Jewish ceremony at 5:00 p.m. About one hundred and fifty people attended, including several of our old friends from Vista. Neither Sara's mother or my mother could make the trip. Corbin was in school at Camp Lejeune, North Carolina so he missed it also. My brother, Don, and sister in law, Pat, made it, as did Sara's half-brother, John, and his wife, Martha Lou. Darby did a wonderful job helping Amy get everything organized. I knew that Sara would have loved to help organize her daughter's wedding. Though now she was just a silent observer. When people would ask her how she was doing, she just smiled and said she was fine.

She had a fair time at the wedding dinner. Sara danced with me, then with Marc and later with her brother John. She appeared to enjoy herself, although she seemed fragile.

At about 9:00 p.m. she looked at me and said, "It's time to go back to the motel." She looked tired, so we left long before all the festivities were over. The important thing was that for the time we were there, she appeared to have a good time.

Sunday morning we had breakfast with her brother John and his wife. When it was time to leave, Sara gave John a big hug and then looked as if she were on the verge of crying. She said nothing though. We drove home and Sara did not say a word on the way either. I'm noticing more and more that Sara does not originate conversations. She often does not answer when people speak to her. Her communication is getting less and less.

On May 25 while driving home, I passed Sara driving toward the park and the tennis courts. A few minutes later she returned home. I asked, "Where have you been?" She did not answer, so I asked her again, "Where did you go?" She finally said, "I went to the bank." I was curious so I asked, "Which bank?" She replied, "Our bank." Then she went into the living room talking as she went, "I also went to see the new library." Knowing the library is under construction, I asked, "How does it look?" Sara replied, "Beautiful." More and more I notice Sara makes up answers to questions I ask. In the amount of time she was gone, she could not have gone either to the bank or the new library location and return home. I chose not to challenge her, just listened to answers I knew weren't true.

I knew that soon I would have to figure some way to get the car away from her. Dr. Brown was still registering his concern about her driving. He told me, "Some Alzheimer's victims have, in fact, died when they become disoriented while driving. They end up in remote locations out of gas and lost." I too had read of such incidents. I certainly did not want Sara to be one of those statistics. In just a few days, when I retired, I would handle it.

When I came home, Sara said, "I played tennis this morning." Considering the fact it was raining in the morning, I have to doubt it. Still, her tone of voice was happy, so I didn't question her.

I only had two days to go before I retired. After shaving, I went into the kitchen and could not find Sara. I looked in the garage and her car was gone, which worried me somewhat. She returned shortly and I asked her, "Where have you been?" She said, "To the tennis courts. I wanted to see if anyone was playing?" I just acknowledged her and then went into the garden to do some work.

Then I saw her in the car driving off again. She returned a few minutes later saying, "I just went to the tennis courts to see if anyone was playing."

When I finished in the garden, I went to the store to do some food shopping. On the way home I saw Sara in her car in front of me. When we got home, I asked, "Where did you go this time?" She said the same thing again, "To the tennis courts to see if anyone was playing." That was three times in little over an hour. I asked myself, "How can I let this continue?"

In the afternoon, after returning from Palomar, Sara said, "I want to take a shower." I was definitely for that, as I'd been noticing that her care for personal hygiene was lessening all the time. A few minutes later I went to check to see how she was doing. She said, "I couldn't get the shower to work." Poor Sara, so many things no longer worked for her, and now the shower. I got her undressed and helped her into the shower. Guess I will be doing a lot of this in the future, but at least I will have the time.

Friday, May 27, is my last workday at Palomar. Actually everything is done and the only thing left is graduation in the evening. It will be the first one I've missed in sixteen years, because I am not going.

The next day I took Sara to the lab for her blood work, then we were off for psychological testing. Originally, Dr. White the psychologist, who had done the testing over a year ago, was to do the retesting. However, in talking with Dr. Smith, who handled the scheduling of the retesting I got the impression Dr. White didn't want to do the retest. As I recall, Sara had given Dr. White a lot of grief during the initial testing and apparently she wasn't anxious for a repeat performance. So this time Dr. Green, a clinical psychologist, will do the testing, on two separate days.

When we arrived at Dr. Green's office I had to go through some questions and answers for the doctor. He took Sara into a closed session for the actual testing while I waited outside. Sara left his office twice to come look for me. She wanted to make sure that I wasn't going to leave her. I had to assist her back in each time and encourage her to do what the doctor asked.

Retirement day finally arrived. But it actually feels like nothing has changed. While shaving this morning, Sara took off for the tennis courts. When she returned, without apparently playing any tennis, I gave myself a retirement gift. I took Sara's car keys away from her. I told her, "I'm home now fulltime so I can take care of you. I'll drive you anywhere you want to go." Luckily, she didn't fight me or get upset. I collected all the car keys and hid them. My job was to ensure I had my own car keys under my control at all times.

The day proceeded with Sara asking to go to the tennis courts several times. I kept saying, "I'll take you at your regular time in the morning to play tennis." Each time she would say, "Okay." Then she'd soon return again thinking it was time for her to go to the tennis courts.

As promised, I took Sara to the tennis courts in the morning. We parked and she sat in the car watching. I'd tell her, "Go ahead, get out. I'll sit here and watch you." She wouldn't get out of the car though. She said, "I don't like the people who play on Sundays." So we went home. Throughout the day she would say, "I want to go to the tennis court now." I would tell her, "We've already been there this morning. Tomorrow morning I'll take you again when it's time for you to play." She just says, "Okay."

Monday morning I got up ready to take Sara to tennis. Sara says though, "I don't want to go. I don't like the people who play on Mondays." Later she says, "I want to go to the tennis court." I notice she's not dressed, so I told her, "Go and change into your tennis clothes and I'll take you." She doesn't though, she just goes back in the living room, sits down and watches TV. Then she gets up and repeats the same thing about going to the tennis court, and I repeat my same answer of her changing her clothes and then I'll take her.

I watch her as she gets up, walks into the kitchen, then the bedroom, back to the living room and then sits down and watches TV. After awhile I get used to her routine. There's no argument at least, just repetition which is going to require a lot of patience and compassion. Let's hope I'm up to it!

Chapter 15

Who Was That Man?

*T*hat night I barbecued some pork chops. I went outside to bring in things from the barbecue after we ate. I was wearing my bathing suit, which was a little large. As I was coming in with both hands full, my suit started slipping and I knew if I took a big breath, it would fall off. Sara was following me in the house, and I thought, "Why not go for it?" So I took a big breath and my suit dropped to the floor and I was bare-assed. Sara looked and started laughing! She laughed and laughed! It was the Sara I remembered. For one very brief moment she was back. I must say I really miss the woman I married.

Sara spent three hours on June 1 with Dr. Green taking her final tests. He didn't have much to say when he was done, but he looked a little exasperated. So now I had to wait and see the results. I know they will not be good.

Don and Pat, my brother and sister in law, moved out of their house on June 7 and were heading to their retirement home in Portland, Oregon. Sara and I went over as they finished packing and cleaning up. We waved goodbye as they took off for Oregon.

We started settling into a kind of routine now that I was home fulltime. She doesn't ask to go play tennis anymore and spends most of her days watching TV.

For some reason, she started spending time at our pool table, just knocking the balls around. On occasion she would wash some clothes, some dishes, prune the roses and other plants, and even pick up oranges. There was no consistency though, and nothing I could depend on. I began to pick up all the duties at home, both inside the house, as well as outside. Sara had neglected the inside of the house for some time now, so there was always something I could find to do. I must admit though, I'm sure not much on dusting.

My cooking must be getting pretty good because Sara has put on a few pounds. She is definitely no longer the 110 pounds she maintained for so many years.

Sara was adamant about never gaining over two pounds. All through her life her figure was extremely important to her.

On June 10, Dr. Green called me by phone. He had little to say, just wanted to ask some routine questions regarding Sara, like how she spent her days. He said when he finished his report he would be sending it to Dr. Smith and a copy to Dr. Brown.

The next night I took Sara to the Veterans of Foreign Wars (VFW), where I am a lifetime member. It was a night of dinner and dancing. Sara still responds to music and dances well, even though her ability to speak is lessening all the time. The dinner was a little upsetting, however. After we went through the buffet line, I was leading Sara back to our table, or so I thought. When I got to our table Sara wasn't with me. I went back into the main room and found her sitting at a table with another couple eating her corn on the cob. I said, "There you are. We're over there, at another table." Sara didn't respond though, she just kept eating her corn, as if in a daze. I was somewhat embarrassed and just stood there waiting until she finished her corn. Then I picked up her plate and took her to our table.

We went back to the VFW frequently over the next couple of weeks. Music and dancing was really the only thing I had seen her enjoy in a long while.

June 23, we met with Dr. Smith. Initially it was just I, alone with Dr. Smith. He went over the report from Dr. Green. As expected, sadly, Sara has continued to deteriorate. The highlights of the report, of which I received a copy, included comments such as:

♦ The patient's short-term visual attention span is moderately impaired. . .

♦ Her long-term visual attention is severely impaired. . .

♦ The patient's general cognitive ability ranges from the average to severely impaired.

♦ . . .her attention, conceptualization, and memory are in the moderately to severely impaired range.

♦ The patient's verbal learning ability is severely impaired. . .

♦ The patient's short term verbal memory is in the moderately impaired to severely impaired range. . .

♦ Her long-term verbal memory is severely impaired. . .

♦ The patient's ability in categorization and abstraction is in the severely impaired range. . .

Part of Dr. Green's summary stated: Taken together, the test data suggests diffuse neurological impairment with cognitive dysfunction in the frontal, parietal, temporal and occipital lobes. In comparison with the past test results, the present test results indicate a continued progressive decline of intellectual abilities, especially her memory.

Dr. Green had the following treatment recommendations:

1. It is recommended that Mrs. Ellison be psychiatrically and medically evaluated to determine the medications necessary to manage her disorder with the accompanying behavioral and emotional problems.

2. It is recommended that Mr. Ellison be consulted on and educated about his wife's condition in order for him to reduce the demands placed upon her, and to provide effective visual and verbal cues to facilitate her behaviors.

3. Because of Mrs. Ellison's difficulty in learning and remembering new information, it is recommended changes in her routine be minimized and that if necessary she be provided with information in small, sequential steps with many repetitions.

4. Because of her difficulties in thinking clearly in making good judgments, her life decisions need to be supervised and her behavior needs to be monitored.

Dr. Smith said, "I discussed the report with Dr. Brown on the phone. Both of us agree that Sara should remain on Cognex because it might in fact be helping slow the progress, and I want to prescribe Wellbutrin at 75mg each day. It might help pick her up physically."

Then he said something that I had been thinking about, he thought it was a good idea to get Sara into some kind of adult daycare activities, rather than sitting home all day watching TV. I told him I had explored this idea several weeks ago, but hadn't considered it lately.

I told Dr. Smith, "I took Sara's car keys away from her and now drive her where she wants to go. I offered to take her to play tennis whenever she wanted, but she doesn't want to play anymore."

After our private meeting, he brought Sara into the office. He asked Sara, "How is your tennis going?" She said, "Fine, I play everyday." Dr. Smith asked, "What time did you play this morning?"

Sara replied, "9:00 a.m." Dr. Smith just looked at me. Our appointment had started at 9:00 a.m.

A routine was starting and the next few days are an example: We go out for dinner, or to a movie to which she has no reaction. I get her to take a bath and sometimes she washes some clothes. She will work outside, but won't do it when I am around. I can always tell when she takes her little pruning shears and goes out and cuts some plants or roses. She will cut flowers and makes little arrangements. She wanders around, both inside and outside the house. I ask her, "Is there anything you need?" She always says, "No," then just goes back to watching TV. I do not know why she watches TV, she seems to pay little more than casual attention to what is on. With the children being gone, maybe it's the company that she likes.

June 27, when I was in the pool, Sara came out in her swimming suit and got into the pool. It is the first time since last winter, when I had to ask Dr. Smith to tell her to stop swimming because of the cold weather.

A couple of days later I was getting out of the pool and I heard the doorbell ring. I heard a man talking to Sara, something about tennis. I heard Sara say, "I play everyday." By the time I got dried off and into the house, the man was gone. I asked her who that man was. She just said, "I don't know." I assume it was one of the men from the tennis courts wondering what happened to her. She hasn't played in a couple of months.

As the days passed, Sara really got back into swimming, which is really just kicking around with her paddleboard. But she seemed to like it.

Her planning calendar is basically blank. Just birthdays and such she entered possibly a year ago. She has no activities anymore. Sara's car in the garage causes some problems by its very presence. She wants to drive it, and I have to keep telling her I'll drive her. So I work out a plan. Amy has been using my 1984 Mazda pickup while in college, and ever since she got married. I'd like to get it back because I have some projects planned for which I will need it.

Marc and Amy came down for the Fourth of July weekend. While they were here I traded Sara's 1984 Honda for the pickup. Actually I gave it to them with the title, so it is theirs now. When they left Sara asked, "Where are they going with my car?" I lied one of those white lies, as I said, "They are borrowing it, while I use the pickup." That seemed to satisfy her.

One of the first projects for the pickup was cleaning out the barn and taking stuff to the dump. One of the items to go was Corbin's old unicycle. We had gotten it for him when he was very young. Now it was old, rusted and had a flat tire. I threw it into the back of the pickup with other old stuff. Sara saw it and got it out. She was going to try and ride it. I told her, "You can't, the tire is flat." She tried anyway. When she couldn't ride it, she put it in back into the pickup. However, during the rest of the day and evening, she came back out at least four times that I saw, took it out and tried to ride it. Then she'd put it back in the pickup. It's times like this that I just feel sick. Sara is so ill and there is not one damn thing I can do about it.

On July 9, I barbecued sirloin steak for dinner. Sara started to choke while eating and then vomited. She had a mouthful of meat, but apparently hadn't chewed it before trying to swallow. After cautioning her again, she did the same thing. Then I cut her meat into tiny pieces. Luckily that worked. Looks like another problem developing.

A couple of days later Sara said, "Let's go out for dinner." She has been saying that a lot lately. So we went to San Marcos to one of the many restaurants on restaurant row. We sat down to order dinner. After a few minutes she says, "I'm not hungry. I want to leave, now!" We briefly discussed this, but I finally gave up without eating and went home. When we got home, she still said, I'm not hungry, but I was, so I rummaged around for something to eat.

The Big 5 was still somewhat intact. They still celebrated their birthdays together by going out to lunch. They were aware of Sara's deteriorating condition. One of them called and said, "I'll pick up Sara and take her to lunch with us." So I got her dressed as well as I could. Apparently the luncheon went well or at least no one said anything negative to me about it. Sara didn't say a word about the luncheon when she got home.

In the afternoon, when I was working on my barn cleaning project. Sara would come out of the house to the barn and ask me, "When are we going to the dump again?" We had been there twice in one week. I told her, "When I have a full load." She would go back into the house and a few minutes later come back out and ask me the same question. She must have done this a dozen times. Again it is times like this that make my days extremely long and tiring.

I ordered a new swimming suit for Sara, which she greatly needed. She looked very nice in it and seemed to really like it. I took advantage of the time she was swimming, by washing the clothes she wears everyday now.

I guess Sara's sorority sisters had an annual chain letter that they wrote. On July 24, I picked up the mail from the mailbox, as well as the post office box. There was a large letter from one of Sara's sorority sisters whose name I recognized. The next day I looked around for the letter, but couldn't find it. I looked in the trash and there it was, at least it wasn't torn up. Yes, it was a chain letter with lots of letters enclosed. On behalf of Sara, I wrote a letter for her, explaining what was going on in her life and mailed everything to another sorority sister. I knew she would know what to do with it.

I attended another caregivers meeting on July 25. Not sure why I go, I probably won't much longer. I am more depressed after I attend a meeting than before I go. The only help I see it does for me is to put the present into perspective which looks pretty good in contrast to the bleak future I envision ahead of us.

Chapter 16

Night Becomes Day

*J*n my role as a fulltime caregiver, I'm finding I need some time to myself and also some help with Sara. I had worked hard all my life, always the equivalent to two jobs and sometimes three. It never occurred to me that I couldn't take care of Sara all by myself, that is until I tried it.

Our doctor suggested daycare some time ago, but I still wanted to do it as long as I could. The time had come and I had already done my research. My choice was Tripler's Daycare Center in Oceanside. It was further to drive, but I thought it would be the best for Sara. I had taken Sara for the TB testing as a prerequisite for attending daycare.

I called Bob, the director, and we discussed enrolling Sara in the center, which operated five days a week. He suggested that he come to our home to meet Sara first. He agreed to come for lunch.

On July 29, Bob came to lunch and we visited afterward. He talked about his center and said to Sara, "I think you might enjoy spending part of your day at my center." He went on to describe their activities such as walking, arts and crafts, table tennis and music therapy. He said, "It's something you might enjoy doing instead of just staying home all the time." Sara just smiled and looked at me and said, "I'll go." It would cost $43 per day. None of Sara's old friends ever came to see her anymore, so life at home was not very exciting. It's sad to see Sara with the TV as her only friend now.

August 1 is Sara's first trip to the daycare center. It's open from 9:00 a.m. until 3:30 p.m., which is good, because I can beat the traffic both ways. Sara went into the center willingly with Bob and I left. When I picked her up in the afternoon, Bob wasn't as lighthearted as he had been. He just said, "She had a mediocre day. Her memory is really poor. She did not participate in many of the activities. I think she needs to come often to get into the routine of things."

On the way home I tried to find out from Sara about her day. I asked, "What did you do during the day?" She answered, "We went on walks." Then I asked her, "What did you have for lunch?" She replied, "We had turkey, mashed potatoes and gravy and milk." Later I coaxed Sara to tell me more about her day. Sara said, "Some of the ladies were in such bad shape." Then she started to cry, which made me feel so sorrowful for her. I tried to cheer her up a little and reminded her how much she used to love helping the elderly. I asked her, "Did you try to help any of them?" She said, "I did."

I have talked to Sara's mother fairly often and have had Sara talk to her. Sara's mother often says, "I just can't really believe that Sara is as bad as you describe her. She seems okay when I talk to her. She looks good in the pictures you send me." I thought for awhile, "How can I get Grammy to understand the severity of Sara's condition?" After thinking about it for some time, I asked Grammy, "How would you like to take care of Sara for a few days while I go fishing?" Grammy said, "I'd love to do that. You just bring Sara up to me, and I'll take care of her as long as you want."

Sara and I left for Placerville on August 3. We arrived late in the afternoon and I spent the night. The next morning I got up and was ready to go. As I was trying to leave, Sara acted frightened and said, "I'm coming with you. Don't go off and leave me." That was the beginning. It took a lot of convincing by both Grammy and myself to get Sara to let me out the door. Finally I left and headed for Utah to go fishing. The fishing was good which was really therapeutic for me. For a short time, my mind was off of Sara.

I enjoyed my time with Andy Gilmour, an old friend from Palomar. I really needed the support of a respected friend of many years.

The drive was terrible, though. Road construction all the way! On the way back to Placerville, I switched routes and went through Las Vegas. It was a good stop for me, not like the last time I was there with Sara when she was at the beginning of what I termed, bizarre behavior. I won over $300 at Binions casino in an Omaha game. What can I say, with some good luck in fishing and now some good luck with cards, I felt refreshed. I was ready to go back to my self-appointed job as a fulltime caregiver. Maybe my mood would be helpful to Sara as well.

When I got back to Placerville, Sara's mother was convinced. She said, "I just had no idea how bad it was, until I saw her with my own eyes." Sara had taken ill with a cold. I called a couple of times, but Grammy had just said, "Don't worry. Have a good time fishing. Everything is going as well as it can." Grammy spoke in a disappointed tone as she said, "The only thing she would do was sit and rock in the rocking chair and watch TV." At least Sara acted like she was really glad to see me. She just said, "I just want to go home. Can we leave now?" So we packed up and headed back to Vista. I knew that Grammy wouldn't have any problem believing me in the future when I tell her about Sara's days. I also felt sorry that Grammy had to face the truth about her only daughter.

August 18 was to be a nightmare day! This morning Sara vomited at breakfast. This was not the first morning Sara had vomited at breakfast so I didn't think too much of it. I left and was gone most of the afternoon. Upon returning I happened to look in the trash and found twelve empty cans of Sprite, plus three empty cans of Mountain Dew and fourteen empty containers of fruit/ berry juice! It was just yesterday that I bought a pack of twelve cans of Sprite. Either she drank them or emptied them and threw away the containers. Regardless, I knew, "Something was wrong!" She was throwing up again.

I immediately called Dr. Smith. He said, "Bring her into my office in the morning. In the meantime don't let Sara have anything other than Gatorade to drink."

It's hard to believe that Sara could have consumed that much liquid, but all the containers were empty.

We met with Dr. Smith the next day. He said, "I'm going to prescribe Zoloft, 50mg each day. Also I want to have some blood work done."

> I am having a hard time with Sara and her liquid consumption. Sara seems to have no turn off switch when she drinks. At least, I only have Gatorade for her now.

> August 20, both Darby and Corbin come home for the day. Sara vomits at lunch again. In the afternoon, Darby takes Sara shopping. I tell Darby, "Try to buy some bigger bras for Sara, because she has put on weight." Darby said, "Okay." When they came home, Darby said, "I tried, but Mom refused to cooperate."

On August 23, near as I can determine, she drank three 32-ounce bottles of Gatorade in the morning. We went to see Dr. Smith. He said, "I'm concerned about Sara's body chemistry. If we can't get this straightened out, she could go into seizures. I may need to hospitalize her if things don't improve. I'm going to order continued blood studies to monitor her body chemistry. Let's take her off of the Zoloft and start her on Paxil, 20mg once each day."

Dr. Smith also talked with Bob at the daycare center. Afterward Dr. Smith told me, "I definitely think Sara should participate in his daycare program more often."

When I picked her up in the afternoon, Wednesday, August 24, Francis, one of the personnel said, "She had a real good day. She played table tennis and was clearly the champion. Bring her back this Friday." When we got home Sara said, "I want some Gatorade." I had bought several bottles and hidden them so I could limit her access. I said, "Okay, I'll bring you one bottle." And I did, I brought one 32-ounce into the house. She gulped it down, drinking it before dinner. Fortunately she did not vomit at dinner. I didn't know what to do, except just give her one bottle at a time.

We saw Dr. Smith in the morning, he sent us to the lab for more blood work.

I was watching a football game on TV, Friday, August 26 when Sara went to bed at about 8:30 p.m. and I followed at about 10:00 p.m. Around 10:30 p.m. Sara asked, "Is it time to get up?" I said, "No, it's 10:30 at night. It's time to sleep." Every few minutes she would wake me up and ask once again, "Is it time to get up?" I kept saying, "No!" At around 11:00 p.m. she got up and went into the bathroom. She had not returned after a few minutes so I got up to check on her. She was getting dressed. I said, "Sara, please come back to bed. It's time to sleep, not get up." She refused and said angrily, "You are a son of a bitch." Then she proceeded to hit me. All I could do was restrain her until she quit.

Then she went out to the kitchen and started her usual morning routine, as if it were daylight. Dumbfounded, I just watched her. She opened the garage door and took Spud out. Next she started the coffee maker. Then she went back in our bedroom and even made the bed. Next, she came back to the kitchen and ate her breakfast of fruit, which I prepared each night and left in the refrigerator. I could say nothing to get through to her. To her, it was time to get up and start her day and she started watching TV.

Around midnight, I just gave up. I closed the garage door and went back to bed. I got up a couple of times to see how she was doing and she was just watching TV.

At 3:30 a.m. she came into the bedroom and asked, "Can I come to bed now?" I said of course and she got in bed and went to sleep. At 5:30 a.m. she woke up, and woke me up, asking, "Is it time to get up?" I said, "No, it's time to sleep." She got up anyway, and this time I didn't try to stop her.

This morning I was to take her to the daycare center. Sara said, "I don't want to go. It's too depressing." I reminded her that Dr. Smith wanted her to go. Sara just pouted and said, "I'm not going." She acted very upset. The only way I could have gotten her to go was to forcefully take her, so I decided to just let it be.

I called Dr. Smith immediately and left a message regarding Sara's actions during the night and this morning.

All of this is beginning to make me feel really helpless. I don't know how to deal with what's going on in our lives. And I'm getting tired of feeling this way all the time, I don't know how much more I can take without erupting myself. I don't think I could live with myself if I went out of control and ever hurt Sara, so I have to find better solutions soon.

On Saturday, we went to Dr. Jones for more blood tests. I would think with all the blood tests Sara had taken, that some sort of diagnosis would be forth coming. They are as puzzled as I am, though. They still can't determine why she vomits and drinks so much liquid.

On Sunday, I continued a fence building project in the backyard. I had torn down the old wooden fence and had put up a temporary wire fence so Spud couldn't get out of the backyard. Sara would come out and watch me for awhile. Then she'd go back into the house, then come out again, then back into the house, and out again. She kept asking me over and over again, "Do you want me to help you put up the wire fence?" It wasn't a wire fence I was putting up, but a wooden fence, she couldn't get it so finally I took the roll of wire fence and put it in the barn so it would be out of sight. I was starting to lose my patience. I was getting angry! I was beginning to get scared, as I could not help how I was feeling about her continuous, repetitious questioning.

On Monday I tried again to get her to go to the daycare center, but she said, "I won't go." In the afternoon I went to see Dr. Smith. We discussed all the problems I was having with Sara. He asked, "Do you think you should seek counseling for yourself?" I just said, "I know what my problem is, it's solutions I need. I doubt if counseling will be of much benefit to me. I've already been to support groups and I feel more depressed after I leave. I like the feeling I get when I'm stimulating my mind by playing cards or going fishing, that works better for me." I'm not so sure Dr. Smith agreed with me, but he didn't try to push his opinion.

Finally on September 2, we met with Dr. Jones again. He said, "I'm sorry but we can find nothing physically wrong with Sara. All the blood testing turned up no answers. Just try and more closely monitor her liquid intake and make sure her food is easy to eat." I walked out from Dr. Jones' office somewhat dejected.

September 3, I took Sara to Long Beach to see Amy and Marc.

Monday, September 5 was Labor Day. We went to the movies and saw *Wagons East*. During the movie, Sara said, "I have to go to the bathroom." I thought she would be okay, because she had been there many times before. When she was gone for too long though, I went to look for her. I sent one of the female attendants into the woman's bathroom to look for her, but she wasn't there. I started to get a little panicky. I started looking in the other show rooms. Finally I found her sitting all alone, watching a killer type movie which was nothing like the cowboy movie we had been watching. She acted as if everything was normal. At least I was relieved to find her. I took her by the hand and led her back to our movie. I really couldn't keep my attention on the screen however, as I began to realize I had yet another problem to worry about.

That night, Sara got up at 11:00 p.m. and started her day. I could do nothing to get her back to bed. Finally, I got up and made doubly sure all the doors were locked, for what good that would do, then went back to bed. She stayed up all night, and I barely slept. After a couple more nights of this kind of activity I began to wear out physically.

I can't figure out how Sara keeps going.

She still won't go to daycare. Her routine is to wander around each day in and out of the house, slamming the door behind her. If I am outside, she will come outside and just stand and stare at me, watching me work. She keeps asking me one question over and over until she switches to a new one, which she asks over and over.

I try to feed Sara the right foods, including lots of fruit and vegetables, but she eats anything and everything now. She'll eat whatever is in the refrigerator or cupboard, it's the same as with the drinking of liquid, she has no shut off valve now, she doesn't know when she's full. She doesn't remember that she just ate. She has gained 24 pounds in the last year! If she were mentally well, she would have a fit! If she got a pound over a 110, she would just about stop eating and starve until she was back to 110. I have had to buy a couple of new belts because all her others are too small. It's time to buy her some new clothes again, as everything is way too tight on her now.

We went back to see Dr. Smith on September 12 for a medication check. He asked Sara, "How is your tennis going?" As always she said, "Good, I played this morning." Dr. Smith told Sara, "I think you need to return to the daycare center." She nodded, "Okay." I took her to the daycare center after her doctor appointment and she walked right in with no problem. When I picked her up she just said, "I had a good time."

The next day I took her to the daycare center. The minute we drove out of the driveway she said, "I don't want to go. I don't want to go. I don't want to go," over and over again. I just kept driving and tried to ignore her. When we got to the center she said, "I will not get out of the car." Bob met us and tried to help, but she wouldn't get out. Finally, Bob gave me the keys to his car and said, "Leave, let me handle this." I finally did. I drove around the block, then came back after a few minutes to see what was happening. After about 45 minutes, Bob got Sara out of the car. When I picked her up at 3:15 p.m., she just said, "I had a good time. I'll go back tomorrow."

This past week has not been good. Once she got up and walked around the house and came back to me saying in a panicked tone, "I can't find my mother." I have no idea why she thought her mother was with us. She really thought her mother was there though, that's for sure. Another day she said, "Someone 'black topped' our driveway," as if it had just happened. It had been over eight years since we had our driveway done.

The next visit to the daycare center was met with resistance again. It took Bob over thirty minutes to get her out of the car. He came out with a chair and sat and talked to Sara until she got out. I watched the whole ordeal and said nothing. He told me with some conviction, "It will get better."

On September 17, I found a message from Sara's mother on the answering service. She said, "I called Sara earlier and after talking for just a brief period, Sara just hung up on me." I felt sorry for Grammy, but there was nothing I could do.

Now it is Sara who is exhausted. She fell asleep in her chair while I was watching a football game. She woke up later and started vomiting again, and did so off and on for an hour. . .still no explanation.

The times Sara was in the daycare center, I took the opportunity to do some research for the future. This research involved identifying and visiting various nursing home facilities. The way things were going, I realized I might have to place Sara in a care facility, fulltime, at some point in time. When the time came though, I didn't want to have to make a decision without having looked at all the possible options. I went around North County San Diego to look at the available facilities. I found lots of places, but many would not take Alzheimer's patients. Some would indeed take Alzheimer's patients, but their facilities were not secure, their patients or patrons could just wander off. That concerned me, as wandering was one of the things that already really scared me about Sara. I had to keep my eye on her almost all the time now.

There was an article in the paper about a man who had Alzheimer's wandering off. His wife looked everywhere for him but couldn't find him. He was found after he was dead.

> The way Sara wanders around all the time, especially at night now, I can see one night where she just might wander off and be lost herself. I just can't let that happen to her.

Sara's situation, unlike many of the patients I viewed on my visits, is that she is physically in excellent condition. It's her mind and her feelings that are not in great condition. The years of playing tennis, and the fact she was only 59, make her extremely mobile. If she were in her seventies or eighties I could see she might have somewhat different needs. My concern in looking at facilities was for her physical safety, as much as for her care.

I found two facilities that met my criteria for safety. Both were geared for Alzheimer's patients and were locked facilities where patients could not get out. I had no plans to put Sara in a facility at this time, but I knew the time might not be too far away. I needed to talk with our children. I also wanted them to look at some of the facilities I had found. Darby worked in a nursing home as a volunteer from her sorority while at University of California-Irvine, and had experience with some Alzheimer's patients.

On September 18, I arranged for Darby, Corbin, Amy and Marc to come home for the day. I gave them addresses of two facilities and asked them to please go visit them without me and let me know what they thought about the facilities. As I expected, they did not have a whole lot to say except, "They look okay to us. We'll leave the final decision up to you." I expected them to say that, as the final decision in our household had always been left up to me, that was Sara's choice, "Wait until your dad comes home. He'll make the final decision." Still, this was their mother I was dealing with and I wanted them to be involved in the process as much as possible without burdening them.

The kids had not been here day in and day out and they didn't really know exactly what has been happening to Sara. I could tell them about it, but being part of her day is a different story, as Sara's mother could testify to.

Chapter 17

As Sara Dies, I Cry

*A*fter a couple of days, Sara finally slept a whole night through! Sure makes the next day a little easier to address. One day she asked, "Where is my car?" Although it's been gone for some time now, I can expect her to ask me the same question all day long.

The next couple of weeks turned out to be kind of a roller coaster. She would be up two and three nights straight and then sleep completely through two and three nights. One night she even slept for twelve hours!

> Dr. Smith said, "Give Sara a couple more Haloperidol tablets when she gets up in the night." I wish they would work, but many times they don't. On October 7, Dr. Smith changed Sara's medication and put her on Mellaril at 75mg. It worked nicely for three nights and then that was it. So he upped the dosage to 150mg. That didn't work either.

A week later we went to the movies. She had to go to the bathroom five times in the first forty minutes. I had to go with her for fear she'd wander off outside or into another movie theater. By the time she was through going to the bathroom five times, I just took her home. It's senseless to watch the movie. We'd already lost the continuity of the story.

For some reason Sara has been thinking we are going to see her mother. Don't know where she has gotten this idea, but she keeps talking and asking about it for the next several days. "When are we going to Placerville to see Mother?" over and over and over! There was no way to shut this out of my mind, she needed an answer every time she asked me. To her, it was the first time she asked.

Sara is up almost every night. She has the same routine starting with turning on every light in the house: living room, dining room, kitchen, game room and bathrooms. At least she doesn't go upstairs. I find myself getting angry all the time now. Maybe it's because I am tired all the time. I read a book on Alzheimer's which compared it to a "36 hour day." This was not an exaggeration, but reality. I was starting to feel like a prisoner in our own home. I couldn't go anywhere, as now I couldn't leave Sara alone for even a moment.

Sara started saying, "My food is too hot." She began opening the refrigerator and getting ice cubes out saying, "I've got to put some ice in my coffee and soup. It's too hot." It is not unusual for her to feed Spot, the cat, twice within an hour. She doesn't remember. Needless to say, Spot enjoys it.

November 5 is the day that President Ronald Reagan announced he has joined Sara in the individual battle they face with Alzheimer's. This will no doubt draw a little more public awareness to the disease. I am sure many in the public will be saying to themselves, "What's Alzheimer's?"

I have tried to remember the first time I heard about Alzheimer's. I think it was a simple little newspaper announcement that movie actor Edmond O'Brien had been diagnosed with Alzheimer's. The article was accompanied by a story about Dr. Alois Alzheimer who first described it in 1906. That was many years ago. About the only time I ever heard about it again was when a famous person was noted as having it. The names of such famous figures as Dana Andrews, David Niven, Sugar Ray Robinson, Rita Hayworth and Arlene Francis are on a continually growing list. But Sara, along with a few million others will go unnoticed.

I never heard anyone mention that Alzheimer's was the fourth leading cause of death among adults age 75 to 84, but that would not have helped alert me in figuring out what, at age 57, Sara's problem might be.

Sara is into trying to wear clothes that no longer fit, only because they are familiar, and she's not really interested in the new clothes I buy that fit her.

Sara no longer has any concept of days, dates and time. She can no longer work any of the appliances in the kitchen. She can no longer make coffee. Either there are no coffee grounds, or no water or both, or she doesn't turn it on. Her life is one of total confusion. If she does something right, it probably is more due to luck, than to concentrated attention. Surprisingly she is able to play table tennis at the daycare center when I can get her to go.

One day or I should say night, Sara and I engaged in sex. She was quite excited and the most responsive I could remember. It was almost like our very first time, so many years ago. It was a remarkable evening, but it was to be our last. It felt like "enjoy yourself tonight because it is the last time." After that rather pleasurable evening, all my sexual advances were rebuked. She became like a frightened child and one does not, of course, sexually accost children.

Watching TV became her favorite past time. I do not understand why, possibly the noise keeps her company and she is under no obligation to interact.

> I have to wash her clothes frequently, particularly her underpants. She is going to the bathroom constantly, but more often now in her own pants. On November 23, I decided to take a count. She dirtied seventeen underpants from 5:00 p.m. the previous night until 8:00 a.m. this morning.

Thanksgiving arrived November 24. Darby, Corbin, Amy and Marc all came home. Sara said, "I don't feel really well." She did not look well either. She vomited her dinner, which I'm sure was a turn off for the kids. I took her vomiting in stride, after all I had become used to it. I felt embarrassed for Sara vomiting in front of her children. She went to bed at 7:00 p.m. and slept until 7:00 a.m. I can truly say that night I could give thanks, and the thanks was for a full night of sleep. I was in a state of perpetual tiredness. I really don't know if the kids were aware of what was going on inside of me. I tried to never burden them about myself, even though I was becoming concerned. The next day Sara ate off and on all day. I guess she just can't remember she eats, so when food is out, she eats over and over, just like she asks questions over and over.

We saw Dr. Jones on November 26. We had been to see him a couple of days before Thanksgiving to try and figure out her bathroom problem. He said, "Her urine is fine, but she has a very bad yeast infection." I got pills and lotion to treat her. She spent the day going from bathroom to bathroom. She kept all three of them running one right after another.

> Today Sara said, "I love you." A simple statement, but so nice to hear. I told her, "I'm sorry I can't take better care of you." She slept from 6:30 p.m. until 4:00 a.m. The next three days, she is up all night again, with all the lights on. Finally she says, "My back hurts." It's probably from sleeping in the lounge chair at night in front of the TV. Anyway, I took her to see Dr. Bendher.

The strainer from the kitchen sink was missing. I looked everywhere for it. Finally I accidentally found it in the garage in a bucket where I keep oranges for squeezing. One can only guess how it got there.

Sara celebrated her 59th birthday with a visit from her Big 5 friends. They brought pizza and ice cream. My sister in law, Pat Ellison, joined in, and they all seemed to have a good time. The next day, Sara remembered nothing of her birthday party and asked, "Where did the cards and gifts come from?"

December 14 was the first day in a long time that Sara did not fight my taking her to the daycare center. That was a real relief! It has been a battle from the time we get in the car until we arrived.

We visited a new chiropractor on December 16. Dr. Bendher told us, I think somewhat relieved, that she no longer participated with our insurance carrier. I picked Dr. Wiply, who was much closer to home. He also seemed to understand Sara's situation and was quite caring in his treatment of her, which I greatly appreciated.

Sara started her Christmas a couple of days early. On the night of the December 23, she got up and raided her Christmas stocking. She opened not only her presents, but also some I had for the neighbors. Amazingly, afterward she turned off the lights and came back to bed. It's the first time the lights were not on in the morning in a long time.

Everyone showed up for Christmas and the girls brought their dogs. All of us assisted in putting the dinner together. It was a very nice day. Sara even changed her clothes a few times, trying on her new things. It's certainly nice to have an enjoyable day once in awhile.

The day after Christmas, Corbin, Amy and Marc left, but Darby stayed. She helped take down the Christmas tree and packed everything away. She actually got rid of a lot of old stuff. Sara had collected so much in the way of decorations over the years, its amazing.

December 27 was an uneventful 60th birthday for me. Sara, Darby and I went to the movies. Fortunately Sara didn't ask to go to the bathroom once. That was a birthday present in itself.

On Saturday, December 31, I was watching a football game in the morning on TV, when Sara actually asked, "Can we go to the daycare center now?" It was difficult telling her it was closed on weekends. She begged, "I have some things that I have to do at the center." At least instead of saying, "I don't want to go," over and over, she was now saying, "I want to go." This was a tremendous relief to me. I had felt really terrible making her go, even though Bob had assured me this was the way it would turn out.

During the day she kept telling me, "You have a birthday coming up soon." And I kept telling her, "It was four days ago." She nodded like she understood, and then in a few minutes, she would once again say, "You have a birthday coming up soon." At least, she was sort of jovial when she said it.

For the next few days, Sara slept twelve hours each night. With both of us rested, the days are so much nicer. Then Sara said something new, she said, "My feet hurt." On checking them out, I could see why. I have neglected her toenails and one is in grown. I took her to a podiatrist who did a major job of trimming. Just one more thing I would have to monitor.

Don and Pat were once again visiting for the winter in Oceanside, so on January 13, we stopped off at their place for coffee and then proceeded to see Dr. Smith.

In a recent conversation, I was told that Alzheimer's is not a mental or emotional disease, but rather a physical body disease. A psychiatrist or psychologist may not be the best medical person to handle the condition of an Alzheimer's person.

> As time has passed and I have learned so many things the hard way, I can see where I would do things differently now.

The first thing I should have done was to go to the local Alzheimer's Association and receive guidance and advice. They have a full list of doctors that deal with Alzheimer's, as well as lawyers that are familiar with what to do. They have informational literature available. With the information now obtainable through the Alzheimer's Association, I would have known that what Sara encountered day to day was totally normal for her condition, and not abnormal. I would have known what to expect.

In my case, the doctors were too reluctant to tell me that Sara might have Alzheimer's. I believe they should have at least let me know early on that Alzheimer's was one possibility. I would have known how to help Sara so much better. We started out thinking that Sara was just suffering from depression, menopause, or "empty nest syndrome," which a psychologist or psychiatrist was capable of dealing with through counseling or emotional work. That's not the way it turned out.

After a few good nights, Sara once again started getting up in the middle of the night and commencing her early morning routine. The medication didn't seem to be working. I just wish she would stop letting Spud out at night. We have already lost one dog to the coyotes.

On Saturday, January 14, Sara wanted to go to the daycare center again. She got dressed and said, "I'm ready to go." I told her, "It is a weekend and they are not open." She went out and got in the car three times thinking we were leaving, although I kept telling her, "We are not going." Finally I had to lock the car so she could not get in.

> I did some cleaning and washing today. Also vacuuming. Sara kept following me around saying, "You are doing a good job." She follows me everywhere, even into the bathroom.

On Monday I took her to see Dr. Wiply because she continues to say, "My back is hurting me." After her visit to the chiropractor, I took her to the daycare center where no doubt she would be the table tennis champion again.

Then I made my first venture into the bridge club. Fortunately there were not very many people there. I got my first introduction into duplicate bridge. I always liked cards and I could see immediately that it would stimulate my mind. The director, Ralph, was very understanding and helped me get started. Unfortunately, I had to leave early to pick up Sara. I didn't know I was messing things in the game up so badly by doing so, but I had no choice. I told him my problem. Ralph said, "I understand. I'll work around it if you want to come back." I said I would be back.

I received a telephone message on January 18 from Bob, the director at the daycare center, saying he had quit. I was sure sorry to hear that. He had done so much to get Sara to go to the center and helped in so many ways. I hated to see him leaving. Hopefully this wouldn't adversely affect Sara. I could see already that there was a high turnover in the professional caregiver field. They probably burned out, just like I was doing.

"Good morning, good morning, good morning," was all Sara could say on Saturday, January 22. She asks to go the daycare center between the "Good mornings." I still can't get her to understand it's closed on weekends, but I know enough to lock the car now so she won't get inside and wait. Somewhere in the mix she says, "I think Corbin may become a Marine."

She has had a jacket with a broken zipper that she has been wearing all the time lately. She keeps trying to work the zipper, but it is broken. She can no longer fix it, and neither can I. Finally I get my hands on it and dispose of it. It makes me feel better, and she never even noticed it was gone.

Then, one day, Sara took her rings off and didn't know what fingers to put them back on. She has been taking them off and putting them back on, but this is the first time she didn't know which fingers to put them on. There was a time when Sara would never, ever, take off her wedding ring.

I took Sara to the daycare center on the 25th. She really likes to go now, but then I got a call saying, "Sara is very ill. You'll need to come and pick her up."

After leaving the daycare center I headed for Dr. Jones' office. He wasn't there, but one of his associates, Dr. Oldman, who had seen Sara often over the years, was. He gave Sara a shot for a virus and then got rather blunt about Sara's condition. He said, "If you are willing, I could hospitalize her to clear up this medical condition. Then she could be moved directly into a fulltime nursing facility." He said, "I think it's time to do this. Her condition is not going to improve."

I told him, "I think about it everyday, but just don't have the will or guts to do it." I added, "I'm also not sure, financially, how long I could hold out if I put her into a home." He seemed to understand and just said, "Any time you are ready, give Dr. Jones or me a call."

In my research I found that a doctor has to admit patients to care facilities, you just can't walk in and dump a loved one at the reception desk. I appreciated his candor, but just couldn't do it then.

That night Sara was sick all night with vomiting and diarrhea. We went back to Dr. Jones' office the next day, and again saw Dr. Oldman. For the next three nights Sara slept twelve hours each night. She continued to say, "I still feel ill." She may be ill, but not enough to keep her from following me everywhere I went. This was beginning to drive me crazy, not one moment by myself.

Since I knew that at some point in time I would have to put Sara in a nursing home, I thought it would be a good idea to talk to

Mrs. Killen, the lawyer, who did all the living trust paperwork. I wanted to find out what she might be able to do in the way of long-term care cost considerations.

I called the office in San Diego and found out she had retired and was off skiing in the Alps. I also found out that my case was filed off in some archives somewhere. There was really no one who could, or would, help me. So much for a lawyer and firm that was going to be around for a long time.

Now I was in the market for another lawyer, this time I wanted to find one who was specifically knowledgeable about elderly law and how to offset long-term care. A family member had played golf with a couple, one of whom had been diagnosed with Alzheimer's, the well spouse had gone to a lawyer about the situation and apparently was impressed with the lawyer. I took the recommendation and met with the lawyer I'll call Mr. Miner. He told me he specialized in elder law. I explained in detail my situation with Sara and I told him that in the future I will probably have to place her in a nursing home and when that happened I'd be looking for some kind of assistance with her long-term care costs. I also told him, I'd been attending some seminars on various financial planning subjects. Long-term care insurance had been discussed. However, as Sara is not eligible for long-term care insurance any longer, I wanted help investigating other programs to which she might be entitled.

Mr. Miner said, "I'm sure I can help you obtain whatever long-term care aid might be available either through government agencies such as Social Security, Medicare or Medi-Cal (which is California's version of Medicare). It probably will cost around $1,800 to do all the legal work." I said, "Thanks, I may call you when the need arises."

> We start off February by seeing Dr. Wiply and
> then to her hairdresser. Then back home because
> she suddenly has a diarrhea problem again. It's a
> fulltime job, almost, just washing her panties.

During the day, Sara usually gets a thought set in her mind. Once the thought is there, it is next to impossible to dislodge. Today I really didn't try. Today's thought was, "Vern, I love you." I heard it over and over again and I must admit it made me feel good, at least the first few times. I even gave her a hug or two along the way. I noticed I was crying, which I do a lot now. It's so unlike me to cry. I had friends who died in Vietnam and I didn't cry, even when my father died, I didn't cry. Now as Sara dies, I cry.

Sunday, February 5, I had to lock the car to keep Sara out. Without the daycare center on weekends it's hard on both of us. Monday she is still trying to make coffee, again unsuccessfully. Fortunately it is the only thing she tries to do in the kitchen now. She goes to the bathroom every few minutes. The daycare center people say, "It is the same while she is here. She goes to the bathroom constantly." I washed fifteen of her underpants today. Today she asked me, "Are you going to keep working at Palomar?" It's been nearly ten months since I retired.

She locked me out of the house again on Wednesday. She does this by closing the garage door while I am outside. I have learned the hard way, to carry my keys with me when I go outside now. Today was an, "I love you, Vern," day. I asked her, "Why do you love me?" She just said, "Because, you're special."

On Saturday, she tried to turn on the TV set, but couldn't manage to get the dials to work for her.

I went shopping on Sunday, but was gone less than an hour. When I came home, a whole bottle of sparkling cider was gone, I'm sure Sara drank it. I had my hands full of groceries and I didn't lock the car. She got in immediately and said, "I'm ready, let's go to the daycare center." I finally got her out and locked the car. The rest of the day, she just followed my every footstep. She would sit and stare at me or repeat her thought of the day, "I'm ready, let's go to the daycare center." I get so angry sometimes!

On Friday, February 17, we went to see Dr. Smith, the psychiatrist. He was not particularly happy with my reports about Sara, but then neither was I, which probably showed. He told me that I might want to get a second opinion regarding Sara. I asked what getting a second opinion would achieve. My guess is he was frustrated and just wanted off the case. He knew she already had a second opinion by a psychologist, a third opinion by a neurologist, and more opinions by two family practice doctors, plus series after series of lab tests, MRI, Cat Scan, X-rays, etc.

Dr. Smith definitely was having a problem with her medication. He was not getting good results with the medication he'd been prescribing no matter what drug he changed to or what dosage he prescribed. I wondered if he had forgotten what he told me after her initial series of testing, "Her brain is in a state of deterioration, and there's nothing that can be done about it." I know I don't think I would have made it through all the changes if I hadn't kept remembering his words.

Chapter 18

For Her Own Safety

*M*onday, February 20, was the day I made the decision to put Sara into a nursing home. The night before was spent in so much anger I thought I might physically hurt Sara. There was no way I could let that happen to her.

Sara went to bed at 8:00 p.m., but kept getting up. She would not listen to anything I said, or more appropriately could not remember from second to second. I kept trying to get her back to bed, to no avail. Finally around 10:30 p.m. I went to bed in Darby's room, but every few minutes she would come in to wake me up with the same words, "Hello Vern." After three or four times, I locked the bedroom door, screaming inside of me at her, "You can do what you want. I just give up."

Of course I got up later to see what she was doing. She had every light in the house on, including upstairs! The sliding glass door to the game room was wide open, as was the garage door. Spud was in her basket and actually looked frightened. Poor little dog has been through a lot with Sara.

I finally just gave up and at 5:30 a.m. I decided to start the day. By this time, Sara was fast asleep. I decided that I really could not take it anymore. I had to give up, for Sara's own safety. I was afraid of my own anger, which was becoming too hard to control. I was also frightened she would wander off and I might not find her.

I was beginning to have more compassion for my parent's decision, when I was a child, to put my little brother Paul, into a home. They too said, "It's for his own safety." At that time, I didn't fully understand and just felt devastated. I was getting ready, now, to do the same with thing with Sara. No doubt, I would again feel devastated.

I finally woke Sara at 6:30 a.m. She said, "I want to sleep some more." I said quite firmly, "We must start the day." I took her to the daycare center first and then I called the nursing facility I had already researched and decided was the best for Sara. It was about twenty-five miles from our home in Vista and a hospital was nearby. I called and made an appointment with the admissions director for 8:30 a.m. the next morning. I was told I would have to bring proof of my ability to pay for Sara's care for a minimum of one year.

I called the kids and told them, "I'm going to have to put your mother into a nursing home tomorrow. I just wanted you to know what I'm doing." They didn't have much to say. Darby asked me one question, "Why did it take you so long?"

I met with the Mrs. Simpson, admissions director of the nursing home, on February 21. I gave her the financial information she required. Mrs. Simpson informed me that Sara could only be admitted as a private pay patient, either through private long-term care insurance or personal assets. She could not be accepted as a Medi-Cal patient.

She mentioned that the nursing facility accepted Medi-Cal patients, but not on initial admission. I told her I didn't have private long-term care insurance for Sara and would have to pay out of our personal assets. Sara was definitely not a Medi-Cal patient. And in fact I didn't really understand how Medi-Cal worked.

Mrs. Simpson informed me that it would be necessary that the director of the Alzheimer's facility in the nursing home, as well as Mrs. Simpson, personally evaluate Sara's suitability for admission.

I didn't know exactly what she meant by "suitability." I told her that Sara was presently at the daycare center and would be there until about 3:30 p.m. today. Mrs. Simpson told me she would try to arrange to evaluate Sara that afternoon.

When I picked Sara up at the daycare center at 3:45 p.m., the admissions director and the director of the Alzheimer's facility were both there. They had completed their evaluation and considered Sara a good candidate for their facility.

On Wednesday, I met with the admissions director for two hours to complete all the paperwork necessary for Sara's admittance. I called Dr. Oldman's office and told him, "The time has come. I'm going to put Sara in a nursing home. I'll need you or Dr. Jones to admit her tomorrow."

I called my brother and sister in law, Don and Pat, who were down from Oregon for the winter, to tell them I was putting Sara in a nursing home the next day and asked if I could enlist their help. Of course they were willing to help me. I told them, "Once we leave her at the home, I'm told I cannot visit her for ten days." The ten days was to allow them to orient her to the facility and its operation without distraction.

In the morning, February 23, Sara and I got up after another bad night. Once we had our breakfast, I took her to Don and Pat's for coffee. When we were finished with our coffee, we all got in my car and went for a drive. The nursing home admissions staff was waiting for us when we arrived. The Alzheimer's director, Mrs. Carlson, took Sara with her. I took Don and Pat and showed them around, including Sara's room, which was a private room. The cost for a private room was $124 per day. Most of the rooms were designed for two people, but the only room available to Sara was a private room, so I had no choice. At the same time I signed Sara up for a semi-private room costing $96 per day.

Private rooms were for patients who paid privately out of their assets or through long-term care insurance. Semi-private rooms were for either private pay or Medi-Cal patients.

Don and Pat were quite impressed with the facility, which pleased me, as I had done a lot of research before picking one. We left and went back home to pack clothes for Sara. Pat helped pick out her clothes and marked them with Sara's name. That is something I would be doing a lot of in the future. We went back to the nursing home and put Sara's things in her room and left. I don't think I could have done it without Don and Pat's emotional support. It was quite hard on me.

Shortly after this realization of what can happen in the future, and their orientation to Sara's new life, Don and Pat took out a long-term care insurance policy covering both of them. When terrible things happen so close to home I guess one's planning can be affected.

I called the nursing home the next day to check on Sara. It was my first night of real sleep in months. When they told me, "Sara had been up most of the night," I told myself, "I made the right decision. There are nurses on duty around the clock that can take better care of her, and I don't have to worry about her wandering off."

It was time to call Mr. Miner, the lawyer, and make an appointment. We met and I told him, "I've placed Sara in a nursing home. The costs, not including medical costs are $124 a day." He said, "I can help you obtain financial assistance for her care." Then he explained his fee fully. "I'll need a retainer of $1000, which is nonrefundable. My hourly rate is $175. You'll have to pay telephone time, copying, postage, filing fees, out of pocket expenses, etc." To me, that meant I would be paying a lot. I didn't know what else to do, and he had been recommended. I had no better leads, so I signed the necessary paperwork to start the process.

Mr. Miner gave me forms to fill out to gather the information he said he would need, which entailed all financial information. I could see it was going to take me some time to assemble all that he was asking. It gave me something to do to take my mind off of Sara though, so I began.

Saturday, February 25 was Darby's 30th birthday. All the kids and dogs came home and we went out for dinner.

On Sunday, Darby and Amy went through Sara's things in an effort to get rid of a lifetime worth of items that would no longer be needed.

I bought two large picture frames that had little individual frames inside where you could put pictures. We started going through photographs we thought would be nice to have in Sara's room. Pictures of the kids, Sara, her mother and father, my mother and even the dogs. Marc used the computer to make labels for each picture. The project turned out quite nicely and we were proud of our joint endeavor.

We loaded up the chaise lounge that used to be Sara's father's. She would sit there most of the time at home, and the nursing home said we could put it in her room. We all went to the nursing home and put everything in her room. We couldn't see Sara officially, but actually we did see her, by looking out the window of her room, across the patio into the dining room, where she was participating in activities. The nurse said, "Sara was up most of the night wandering the halls."

Over the next ten days, I would call and check on Sara. Everything was reportedly going okay, except for her sleeping habits and constantly going to the bathroom. Her liquid intake was completely monitored as is just about everything she does or does not do on a daily basis. There was finally enough help to fully look after Sara.

I spent a great deal of time assembling the inventory of financial information Mr. Minor had requested. The information he wanted involved detailed information on all assets, including insurance policies, income information, Social Security information, bank accounts, investment information such as stocks/bonds, mutual funds, vehicles, and even cemetery plots. Absolutely anything that could be considered an asset had to be listed with exact information. I was finally able to assemble and provide all this information to Mr. Minor.

On Sunday, March 12, we were allowed to see Sara. I took Spud with me and met Corbin at the nursing home. Spud barked at everyone, but finally settled down. They encourage families to bring pets. Sara was most happy to see Spud. We sat on the patio. Sara seemed content. I mentioned, "It looks like they are setting up for lunch." Sara almost jumped out of her chair and headed straight for the dining room, right to her table. She knew exactly where she was to sit. I breathed a sigh of relief. I felt much better seeing that she seemed happy. She smiled a lot, not just at us, but at everyone she encountered. I went home with a good feeling in my heart that I had done the right thing after all.

I visited Sara every day for the first couple of weeks. Sometimes I would take Spud. We would walk around outside the nursing home, which is something the patients got to do, sometimes both in the morning and again in the afternoon.

I had lunch a couple of times with her, I paid $5 each time. I noticed just about everyone had a different menu, depending upon their needs and their ability to eat. Some needed help eating and there were nurse's assistants that helped feed the patients. When Sara was served, her name was on the tray. One day we had baked fish, mashed potatoes, peas, muffin, carrot and raisin salad, milk and ice cream with strawberry topping. If they keep her on this kind of diet three times a day, plus the snacks they get, Sara is going to have an even worse weight problem. I probably worry way too much about her weight, but since it was so important to her throughout her life, I feel somehow responsible to ensure it doesn't increase. I guess now I feel it's up to me to ensure she doesn't gain more than the two pounds she would never let herself gain.

March 28, I took Sara out of the nursing home and back to Vista for a hair appointment. Then we had lunch at the Jack in the Box, because Sara wanted a burger.

On March 29, I drove down to Kearny Mesa for a seminar sponsored by the San Diego Alzheimer's Association. The seminar covered legal and financial concerns for Alzheimer's victims and their family. I was surprised by the large turnout. I picked up a lot of good information. This would be just one of several seminars I would attend in the future, all dealing with legal questions, financial concerns, living trusts, long-term care programs and just about all other aspects of estate planning. I certainly wished I had known all the things I was learning, before Sara started becoming ill.

Sara began saying, "My back hurts." So I took her to see Dr. Wiply who showed a sincere interest in her case. After a couple of weeks, Sara started being tired all the time and quit participating in the activities that she usually did. I took her to see Dr. Smith. The nursing home only administered medications, they did not prescribe, but the nurses had listed their observations. As always Dr. Smith asked Sara about her tennis. As usual, Sara said, "I played this morning." Dr. Smith reduced Sara's Mellaril by ten percent.

Our 33rd wedding anniversary was April 14. I took her a card and an Easter Lily. She opened the card, looked at it and then laid it down. She didn't even try to read it, which saddened me. I found out she could not keep the Easter Lily in her room, I had to deliver it to the nurse's station where all fresh flowers went.

I took Sara out for lunch in Del Mar and found out for the first time that I had to sign her out. I had taken her out before and no one had said anything. We had a big bowl of clam chowder and sourdough bread that Sara loves. She had two "Shirley Temples," and a hot apple crisp with ice cream. Sara could see a Denny's restaurant across the street. As she was eating her lunch, she kept asking, "Can we go to Denny's and have a burger?" Then later she said, "I'm through. Can we go to Denny's now?" I said, "No, but another time." On the way back to the nursing home, we passed a McDonalds, Carl's Jr. and Burger King. At each one, she said, "Can we stop and get a burger?" Regardless, we had a nice time. The constant repetition didn't even get to me since I was only with her for a short time.

> After thirty-three years of marriage, Sara said, "I love you." Although she did not understand what day it was, or how long we had been married, she did say, "I love you," which made it all somehow worthwhile. My anger had dissipated soon after I put Sara in the home and I could experience my love for her again.

Sara's wristwatch was missing. I reported this to the nurses, but it was never to be found. I had to take Sara's earrings away, she kept pulling on them causing an infection and bleeding.

All the kids and dogs showed up Easter Sunday. We all went to see Sara. Darby prepared an Easter basket full of candy for Sara. She ate most of it and Corbin finished the rest. Sara's two thoughts for the day were "What is Spud doing?" and "Can we go for dinner at the Casa Linda?"

The next day, April 17, I took a break and went to Oregon to see my family for a week. I stopped off in Placerville to see Sara's mother and I gave her pictures of Sara. Then I was on to Oregon to see my mother and sister in Corvallis, then Don and Pat in Portland, along with their kids and families. It was the first time I had visited my family without Sara. This time I actually got to enjoy them without having to worry about what she would say or do. Still though, I missed Sara being by my side. I was in a period of adjusting to what it was like to be totally alone all the time.

I got home on the 25th, just in time for Corbin's 29th birthday. He stayed in the house while I was gone and took care of the dog and cat.

When I visited Sara after my trip, she seemed happy to see me. I showed her pictures of our anniversary luncheon and of her mother. Initially she didn't recognize her mother, but with some prompting, she remembered. I put the pictures back in my shirt pocket. A short time later she saw the pictures and said, "Oh you have some pictures! Let me see them." She took them out and looked at them as if she had never seen them before.

As Mr. Minor continued to work on Sara's application for government assistance, I continued the private pay for Sara's care. She had finally been moved into a semi-private room at $96 per day. Based on a review of my financial inventory that I had given Mr. Minor, I would be able sustain Sara's care for about three years. After that, if Sara could not qualify for Medi-Cal or some other program, I was not sure what I would do. We had tried to be responsible, invested and put up savings so we could take care of ourselves in our later years. Surely I wouldn't ever end up like my father, who during the depression, often worked for food to put on our table. Or would I? With the laws continually changing, the Constitution being interpreted differently by the courts, who knows what tomorrow will bring?

Chapter 19

Wedding Rings Come Off

O ne day we were sitting in Sara's room and she was asking her usual question "Where's Spud?" She then pointed to a room across the hall and she said, "That is my other room." I looked puzzled and asked, "What do you mean, you have another room?" She got up, proceeded to go across to the other room and opened the clothes closet. It seemed to make Sara happy. I guess it didn't hurt anything, although I would have felt personally better if there had been more control of the patient's clothes.

As time moved along, I was becoming less impressed with Mr. Minor's knowledge of the Medi-Cal application procedures and requirements. One of the initial things I had to do was go to the county social services office to obtain the necessary application forms for Medi-Cal. Mr. Minor told me which office to go to. I would be required to attend an orientation before obtaining the necessary paper work. Mr. Minor sent me to the wrong office. As I learned more, I could see he not only was not knowledgeable about what office to go to, he was not very knowledge about the procedures or requirements.

Although I had retained Mr. Minor to work on Sara's Medi-Cal application, I continued to attend various seminars on the subject of long-term care, living trusts, Medi-Cal, Medicare and various other subjects related to financial and medical planning.

I found there are a variety of entitlement programs available from the government that we are entitled to, but not to expect a nursing home or the state to inform you about them. I would have to learn the process and the rules. Sara had not worked enough to be eligible for Social Security, but at age 62, would be eligible under mine. However, she was entitled to Medi-Cal under the Medicare Catastrophic Coverage Act. Also under this act, Medi-Cal could not impoverish or cause undue financial hardship to myself. That was a relief.

It was at one of these seminars, presented at a local hospital, that I was to meet a Medi-Cal consultant, Mr. Steven H. Gallup. The seminar had the usual presentations on long-term care insurance, living trusts, etc. As part of the presentation, Mr. Gallup gave his talk on the requirements for Medi-Cal qualification. After his presentation, I decided to leave, because I had heard the next speaker on the agenda.

As I was leaving, Mr. Gallup struck up a conversation with me. He said, "I noticed you asked some very specific questions of a couple of the speakers. I'm not sure you got the answers you were looking for." I told Mr. Gallup, "I'm presently working with a lawyer on an application for Medi-Cal for my wife who is in a nursing home. I'm not particularly happy with how things are going with the application procedures, which is the reason I attend these seminars. I am trying to learn more about the process from different perspectives, so I am better equipped."

Mr. Gallup said, "My expertise is entirely with Medi-Cal procedures. Before going into the private sector, I worked for the county social services department and handled Medi-Cal applications." I reminded him, "I'm working with a lawyer, but if things don't move along a little more smoothly, I just might give you a call." I took his business card and left.

Sara is very big on the Hokey Pokey, which she likes to sing and dance to. Strange, she doesn't speak many words, but can sing a whole song.

I have been playing duplicate bridge for the past few weeks on Monday afternoons. It gives me a lot more relief than the support groups I attended. There were different members whose spouses or parents were in nursing homes. When I first started playing I would get paired off with different partners. The last month I have played with the same woman, Mary. We seem to be doing pretty well together. We have come in 4th, 6th, 2nd and finally 1st.

I told Mary about Sara, at which time she told me about her mother in law. Her mother in law has Alzheimer's. She took care of her for three years, until recently, when she and her husband put her in a home. She said, "My mother in law, who is eighty-five, has not recognized either of us for over a year. I am surprised to hear how young Sara is."

On June 14, I flew back east to Washington, DC to attend another one of my Marine Corps basic officers class reunions. I wasn't sure if this would be the last one or not. This one was in honor of the Commandant of the Marine Corps, who was retiring after some thirty-eight years on active duty. He and I had both served in the same rifle company, when we landed in Beirut, Lebanon on July 15, 1958. As usual, many old friends were there with over three hundred husbands and wives in attendance. Many inquired about Sara, noticing she had not attended this reunion. I found out that bad news travels fast.

When I got back to San Diego, on my way home I stopped and saw Sara. She seemed unaware that she had not seen me in four days. She seemed quite happy and was smiling, as always. She asked about Spud and what I was doing? She was just finishing her lunch and had cleaned her plate. She is really putting on weight.

Amy was pregnant and due to have her baby June 19, but the baby hadn't arrived yet. I told Sara the news. Sara seemed concerned and said, "I don't think Amy should be having a baby." In other times, Sara would have been ecstatic knowing she would be a grandmother.

I took Sara to the dentist on June 22. He said her teeth were in bad shape and that she had a cavity. Sara's teeth were always in such good condition and now they were terrible. I told him she had been in a nursing home for the past four months since her last visit. Her teeth were cleaned and an appointment was made to take care of the cavity. The dentist wrote a note for the nurses regarding Sara's need for better dental care. He was rather explicit.

My visits with Sara continue to be pleasant. One day she tried to be funny by making noises and moving her lips and mouth. She was actually funny. She still smiles and actually laughs on occasion. She keeps saying, "I love you," and, "You are special." She will sometimes ask, "How can I get out of here?" She doesn't actually ask to go home, but I know that is what she means. She never misses asking about Spud. One day she asked me how things were going in the Marine Corps. It's been eighteen years since I retired.

Saturday, July 1, I was getting ready to visit Sara, when I found a phone message from Marc. Amy was to have a "C" section at 5:00 p.m. I headed to Long Beach. Our first grandchild, Kyle Tristan Prager, was delivered at 5:34 p.m. This would be just one of many events that Sara would miss and would have loved so much to be part of. I took videos and pictures.

The next day I arranged with the nursing home to show the videos to Sara. Sara had no idea what was going on or that she was now a grandmother. A couple of days later I showed Sara the photos of Amy and Kyle. She understands who Amy is, but can't figure out what Kyle is all about. It was at least a week before Sara finally could remember Kyle's name without help.

When visiting Sara I will often find her asleep in a chair, which means she had been up during the night. One day I found her with mismatched socks on and her trousers on backwards. The attendants try to let those that can, and Sara still can, put on their own clothes in the mornings. I suggested a little more supervision.

July 19 I took Sara to see Dr. Smith. He made no change in her medication. She is on Mellaril 110mg, Zoloft 100mg, and Artane 2mg in addition to her Premarin and Provera. We stopped and had lunch at the Jack in the Box, where she got to have her burger. As always, when she sees babies and little children on our drives she gets excited. She has always loved little children.

The next few weeks were relatively peaceful. Sara talked about Spud all the time. Once she said, "I just gave Spud a bath." Another time, "Spud went to the bathroom in the house," and best of all, "I love you."

> I take her out for lunch a couple of times to the Boll Weevil, where she gets her burger and a handmade chocolate milkshake.

After nearly seven months of working with Mr. Miner on submitting a Medi-Cal application for Sara, it seemed we were getting nowhere. I know he was very good with his monthly legal bills, he was excellent down to the last detail, including billing me for leaving messages on message machines. After nearly $1,800, I was not enthralled with the results. One time he even called me from a seminar he was attending telling me not to send in some paper work I had just completed, he had just learned something different than what he had instructed me to do earlier.

In mid-August I went to Panquich, Utah with a friend from Palomar to meet with Andy Gilmour, who had retired from Palomar College in May. We had a great time and caught a lot of fish.

When I returned, Sara didn't notice that I had been gone for six days. I noted that Kyle's picture was missing from Sara's room and reported it to the nurses. After a couple of days it turned up in her room again.

Sara says some of the strangest things. She has been telling some of the employees, "Vern's a football coach." Not only that, she told me, "I have to wash the windows in the cafeteria everyday." She told me that Amy was putting "double diapers" on Kyle. Then she asked, "How are things at Camp Pendleton?" She just seems to have random thoughts about our past years together, as well as making up things that aren't the least bit true.

I took her to a hair appointment in Vista and had her nails done also. Afterward we went to a local restaurant where she had her burger. She saw a woman who was overweight and said the woman sure was fat. I asked her, "Sara, how much do you weigh?"

She said, as always, "110 pounds." On September 21 she weighed in at 153 pounds. For some reason I am feeling depressed today.

I talked to the director of the Alzheimer's unit regarding Sara's diet and weight gain. She replied somewhat defensively, "I like my patients fat because when they become ill, and they do, they often lose significant amounts of weight. I'm speaking from a lot of experience."

It was during the Medi-Cal application process, that Mr. Minor informed me that I had to apply to Social Security before I could continue the Medi-Cal application procedures. This caused a further delay in the application process. On September 26 I talked with the local Social Security office regarding an application I had submitted for disability in Sara's case. The caseworker indicated that Sara was going to be denied Social Security disability and Supplemental Security Income (SSI).

I informed Mr. Miner to stop the application process until further notification.

Amy and Kyle came to visit Sara on September 29. Sara got to feed Kyle and seemed to have a really good time doing it. She knew exactly what she was doing and needed little direction.

It came to the point on October 1, that I had to take Sara's wedding ring away from her. For some weeks now she has had problems with getting her finger infected because she doesn't dry her hands properly after washing. She has had her ring switched back and forth between hands to try and help. Today, because of her weight gain and the infection, it was almost impossible to get the ring off. So today I had to keep it, until such time she loses enough weight, but then it might still cause her continuous problems. Another day I am not feeling good about the world.

For the first time in a long time, Sara mentioned "Lucy." She asked if Lucy was still outside? She still can't comprehend that Lucy is dead.

Corbin came down on the 10th to visit with Sara. Sara said about herself, "I had to do some filing work in the nurse's office. Also I need $10 to pay for my lunch." She is quite serious when she makes these statements, as if she fully believes them. She keeps going to the bathroom a lot when I visit.

After thinking about it for a few weeks, I decided I would contact Mr. Gallup, the Medi-Cal consultant, and see if in fact he could provide the necessary assistance that I needed to submit a Medi-Cal application. We met for a preliminary meeting in which he explained what he would, and could, do for me, and specifically what I would have to do in the process. He said his fee was a flat $1,000 to handle the application process from start to finish. His confidence and step by step explanation of the process required, convinced me to employ his services. He said he would draw up a service agreement for my signature.

On October 14, Sara kept going to the bathroom again while I was there. One of the nurses said, "We've discovered blood in her panties and have called the doctor." The nurse asked, "Has Sara ever had an hysterectomy?" I replied, "No." While I was there, the doctor had not called back so asked them to please call me at home if there are any problems.

Sunday, October 15, Corbin and I drove up to Monterey Park for a going away party for Darby and her fiancé. Darby, who was now engaged, and her fiancé, were being given a going away party by her fiancé's parents. Amy and Marc came, as did a number of other friends. Darby's fiancé had accepted a job in the computer industry in the Portland, Oregon area and Darby was quitting her job at the Bren Events Center, at the University of California-Irvine, to go with him.

Corbin and I got back to Vista at about 7:30 p.m. As I got out of the car I had an instant headache. Corbin took off to his apartment and I went in the house only to find a phone message from the nursing home. By this time I was feeling chilled and started shaking. I returned the call to the nursing home and the duty nurse said, "Dr. Newhous [who had taken over Sara's case from Dr. Oldman a few months before] has seen Sara and said she has a prolapsed rectum."

I was feeling poorly all night, with chills and fever. I felt a little better in the morning and went to see Dr. Newhous about Sara. He suggested I get a second opinion from a surgeon on Sara's condition. I said I would arrange for that.

On Tuesday, Sara and I were supposed to have a portrait done of us together, but I was feeling terrible, I just couldn't make it. They went ahead and did one of Sara anyway. They had her dressed in an old sweater with a hole in the sleeve, I must say, though, she looked beautiful.

At about 2:30 a.m. Wednesday morning, I went into some sort of convulsions. I was freezing and shaking so badly at times I could hardly breath. I actually had the thought, "I may be dying." It stopped after about an hour and I managed to get in to see Dr. Jones in the morning. The doctor told me I had pneumonia. He shot me full of penicillin and gave me prescriptions for other drugs. I spent all day Thursday hardly able to move, but was able to eat. Finally, by Saturday I almost felt alive again. I knew as soon as I could, I needed to get that second opinion for Sara's condition.

Chapter 20

When I Die

Sara's friends in The Big 5 group had arranged a party in Carlsbad and called to ask me if I could bring Sara. I said I would. I picked up Sara and took her to the party, where The Big 5 leadership had hired a limousine for them to take a ride around the coast area. Sara joined her friends and they took off on their ride. Sara seemed to enjoy the ride. We did not stay at the party long, because she kept wandering off and she showed no interest in the activities. I was pleased they asked Sara to come.

When we got back to the nursing home, Sara said, "My bottom hurts." The nurse checked, and told me, "Sara has rectal bleeding." Finally, on October 26, I got Sara in for an appointment with Dr. Gold, who was a well regarded surgeon. Dr. Newhous had recommended him, but I also checked him out with a retired doctor at the bridge club. Sara became very anxious and confused when the doctor was over an hour late for our appointment, she just wanted to leave.

When the doctor finally tried to examine her, Sara was completely uncooperative and I actually couldn't blame her. He said, "I'm unable to distinguish a problem. All I can do is suggest the nurses keep observing her." It was a very lousy day!

I took Spud with me to see Sara on the October 28. We were sitting together, when she said, "What is Spud doing today?" I told her, "Spud is lying right at your feet." She looked at Spud, but said nothing. I noticed that Kyle's picture, which had been missing again, had returned. I checked Sara's drawers and all the new panties and bras I had recently bought were gone. I reported this to the nurses and said, "I would like some sort of action to turn up her clothing." Many times Sara still showed up at the door in clothes other than hers.

Sara kept saying, "My leg hurts." I reported this to the nurses. The next day I got a call from a nurse telling me, "Sara's leg problem is Cellulitis and Dr. Newhous is prescribing antibiotics."

On Tuesday, October 31, I brought Sara three new panties and a pink robe. We took off to see Dr. Smith for a medication check. He took Sara off of Mellaril and put her on a new drug.

On the morning of November 2, I met with Mr. Gallup and signed a service agreement. At that time he provided me a "Four Phases of Medi-Cal Case Management" outline. Medi-Cal in California is equivalent to Medicaid in other states. There are two arms of Medi-Cal, one for those in poverty, needing assistance such as food stamps. The second arm has to do with catastrophic illnesses or accidents, which is what Sara's condition fell under. He discussed in detail how each phase had to be accomplished and what I would have to do, and in turn what he would do. I felt confident with him.

At least I would not be destitute, which is what could have happened if I had to continue to pay for Sara's nursing home expenses from our savings. I would, in all probability have had to sell our house. This way, at least I would be able to live in the house until I died.

I must admit, I had really mixed feelings. It's not that it wasn't fair, but it was hard for me to think of our home going to the state, and not to our children or grandchildren. Right now, there was nothing I could do about it, but accept the fact that's the way it was. I could tell though, it was one of those things that wasn't going to leave my mind, particularly when the state sent me a letter each year reminding me. You can imagine how it might feel to open your mailbox once a year to find a notice that reads:

"FOR YOUR INFORMATION ONLY

Pursuant to California legislation enacted in 1981, and subsequent amendments in federal and state law, Medi-Cal benefits received by a beneficiary from age 55 are recoverable after death under certain circumstances. Claims are filed against the estate of a deceased Medi-Cal beneficiary and reimbursement is due from the estate or distributee(s). The Department of Health Services (Department) may not file a claim during the lifetime of a surviving spouse; when there is a deceased beneficiary's child who is under age 21, a son or daughter who is blind, or a son or daughter who is permanently and totally disabled. When the surviving spouse of a deceased Medi-Cal beneficiary dies, Medi-Cal may bill the estate of the surviving spouse for either the amount paid by Medi-Cal on behalf of the predeceased spouse or the value of the assets received by the surviving spouse, whichever is less.

Written notice of the death of a Medi-Cal beneficiary, with a copy of the death certificate, is required to be given to the Department at Post Office Box 2471, Sacramento CA 95812-2471. Notice to the county or Social Security does not satisfy this requirement. Reference: Sections 215, 9202, and 9203 of the Probate Code and Section 14009.5 of the Welfare and Institutions Code. For further information, please contact the Department's Estate Recovery Unit at (916)323-4836."

One day I hope to figure something out.

I would be able to keep my car, household goods, personal property and IRA's. I could have no more than a total of $75,000 in assets whether it was in cash, savings accounts, CD's, money market accounts, stocks and bonds, mutual funds, and cash value of life insurance over $1,500. Anything over the $75,000 would not be exempt. The laws change, and did change, so to offer any advice on today's criteria would not be appropriate.

In the afternoon after meeting with Mr. Gallup, I found Sara feeling better about her leg. She really can no longer readily describe when she has a physical problem except to say, "I hurt." While we were in her room she said, "My pants are wet." They were. She said, "I have to go to the bathroom." So I took her. When she sat down, I checked her panties and they were wet and full of defecation. When she was through, she started to pull her panties back up. She was oblivious to her situation. I got her panties off and cleaned her up and got her a new clean pair. I am beginning to think Sara is becoming incontinent, like so many around her. I took her to the nurses, who said, "This is the first time something like this has happened." I doubted it. When I left, I felt sick.

Sara and I had our pictures taken together the next day to make up for the time I had pneumonia and couldn't make it. I brought Sara her pearls to wear and she looked really nice. Unfortunately the photos were poor, so I passed on buying them.

On November 4, the evidence of Sara's situation finally surfaced. One of the nurses called me and said, "While giving Sara a shower, we were able to take two Polaroid pictures of a very pronounced prolapsed rectum. The protrusion is about two inches and extremely red. I have one photo for our files and one you can take to Dr. Gold or Dr. Newhous."

The next day, a Sunday, Corbin, Amy, Marc, Kyle and I, all visited Sara. Kyle was a lot of fun making all kinds of good noises. Sara was not feeling well, but seemed to enjoy our visit the best she could. On Monday, I took the Polaroid photo of Sara to Dr. Gold's office. He wasn't in, so I gave it to one of his nurses, who said she would give it to the doctor and have the doctor call me.

Tuesday, I met with Dr. Gold to discuss Sara's situation. I told him, "Sara could not speak well enough to explain her condition." Dr. Gold replied, "Some people can live with a prolapsed rectum problem, but undoubtedly in Sara's case it will continue to worsen, as she is not competent enough to take care of herself in this situation."

I said, "Based on Dr. Newhous' and the nurse's observations, and observation of the photo, I believe a operation would be necessary." Dr. Gold told me, "It will be a major operation and require Sara to be in the hospital for five to seven days. The operation will require my going in through the abdominal area and doing the necessary surgery. The operation will take out the excessive colon. Then other surgical procedures will be done to prevent the situation from happening again."

He further explained that in preparation for the operation, Sara will need to take certain medications and laxatives to clean out the colon a couple of days prior to the procedure. If I were agreeable, he said the time frame would be in the next couple of weeks. I told him that I believed the sooner the better. He said, "I'll have someone call you when the schedule is finalized."

Sara's condition suddenly worsened. On Wednesday, November 8, Sara was in pain and great discomfort. She had been shaking, vomiting and was in overall distress. The nurses said, "We've talked to both Dr. Newhous and Dr. Gold who are considering getting Sara to the hospital on an emergency basis for the operation." Dr. Newhous was to see her that night with the idea of trying to get her admitted. Dr. Newhous called me at home and said, "Take Sara to the hospital in the morning, for admittance at noon."

Thursday, November 9, I picked Sara up at 11:00 a.m. to take her to the hospital. When we arrived, we were told there were no beds available at the moment. This necessitated Sara being admitted through the emergency room. We waited for three hours. Sara was very upset and hard to control during the wait. Finally a bed became available and I took Sara to her room. The nurses immediately started her pre-operation procedures.

On Friday the pre-operation procedures continued. She was feeling poorly and just wanted out of the hospital. They had her strapped to the bed so she could not escape. Corbin came to visit at around noon. I met with Dr. Gold and signed release forms for Sara. He said, "The operation will take place tomorrow morning at 9:30 a.m. and will last about two hours. Dr. Newhous is going to assist." What was there to say, I guess you don't have to be a surgeon to assist one.

> Today is the 220th birthday of the U. S. Marine Corps. I can remember Sara and I having some wonderful times at the annual birthday balls. Not this year.

Saturday, I got to the hospital at 8:30 a.m. At 9:00 a.m. I helped the nurse wheel Sara to the operating room. Then I just waited. At about 12 noon, Dr. Gold and Dr. Newhous appeared in the waiting room. Dr. Gold said, "The operation went as planned. Sara will be in the hospital for five to seven days and must be on a liquid diet for the next two weeks." At 2:30 p.m. Sara was returned to her room, which was about the same time Corbin appeared. When she saw Corbin, she smiled. She was really doped up.

Sunday morning Sara couldn't say much, except, "My leg hurts." She had tubes in arms and nose, just like on the TV shows. The nurse gave her some pain killing medication through her IV. Sara dozed off to sleep.

Two of Sara's Big 5 friends visited twice over the next three days. On November 14, Sara was able to sit up in a chair for a long period of time. She was mostly quiet.

By November 15 she was looking a lot better, but was still quiet. Surprisingly she did not asked once about Spud.

On Thursday, November 16, Sara was released from the hospital at 1:35 p.m. I drove her back to the nursing home where everyone was glad to see her. I gave the nurses all the orders from Dr. Gold, stressing the fact she could have no solid food, until the doctor said it would be okay.

> On Friday, Sara was not in her room and I had to search for her. I found her asleep in someone else's room. She could only whisper when she tried to talk. She looked very tired, but she wanted to do the Hokey Pokey for me.

Things picked up on Saturday. Sara did some coloring during activity time and seemed very happy. She did her Hokey Pokey with more enthusiasm. Once again she said, "I love you," and, "You are special."

Sunday was the happiest I had seen Sara in weeks! She did a very lively Hokey Pokey, smiling all the time. But she still would go to the bathroom frequently, possibly out of habit, or as a result of her liquid diet.

A former next door neighbor called me to see how Sara was doing. When I mentioned the call to Sara, she had no idea who I was talking about. As on most days when I visited Sara, she said, "I love you Vern." This day I found Sara wearing a necklace I didn't recognize. When I asked where she had gotten it, she said she made it, which of course was not the case. I wondered who she had "borrowed" it from. The nurses must have a real nightmare trying to keep up with the personal belongings of the patients.

On November 22 I found Sara asleep in a chair. When I woke her up, she smiled and got up to do the Hokey Pokey for me. A nurse came and changed Sara's bandage. I watched the process and finally saw the results of the operation, which was a large incision running vertically down her abdomen, closed by forty-one staples. As the nurse was in the middle of the bandaging, the fire alarm went off. The nurse hurried up the bandaging, saying, "I have to get to my station. When the fire alarm goes off, all the locked doors to the facility become unlocked and the patients can get out." It turned out to be just a fire drill conducted by the fire department.

On Thanksgiving Day, I visited Sara in the morning. She said, "I love you Vern," but that is all she seemed to be able to say. I had thought about taking Sara home for Thanksgiving, but I wasn't sure it would be a good idea to have her around a lot of solid food with her being on a liquid diet. I also had reservations about having her home, it might be upsetting to her. Amy, Marc, Kyle and Corbin came home in the afternoon.

The next day we went to visit Sara. One of the duty nurses told us it was time to remove the staples. Amy and I held onto Sara as the nurse took out the staples. A few times Sara seemed to have some pain, but didn't cry or call out.

Sunday was toenail cutting day. I hadn't done it for some time and they were certainly in need of a good trimming.

The chaise lounge we had taken for Sara when she was first admitted, apparently was causing some obstruction problems in her room and she never seemed to use it, although I would often find other patients on it, usually asleep. So, on December 3, Corbin came down and we loaded it up to take back home.

After working for the past four weeks on the Medi-Cal application and supporting documentation, Mr. Gallup came by on December 4 to check over my work. He had a couple of corrections and additions for me to make, but otherwise he said, "Everything looks fine. I'll make an appointment with the county social services for the next week, at which time we will both meet to present the initial application."

I was really grateful for Mr. Gallup's knowledge of government entitlements that we have all paid into for many years. They are available, it's just knowing someone that can take you through the system, as it's terribly complicated. It would be like dealing with the IRS by yourself and not knowing all the rules and regulations.

Sara turned 60, on December 9. Amy and Corbin came to visit. We all went out for lunch at the Boll Weevil, where Sara had her usual burger and chocolate milkshake. We returned to the nursing home with a birthday cake and presents. Sara's mother had sent her a ceramic Christmas tree, which was actually a windup music box. It must have weighed close to 10 pounds! It was a very nice art piece, I guess that is why it disappeared in less than a week, never to be found.

It has become apparent to me that you don't give Sara really nice things anymore. Nice clothes don't last too long, because most are not designed to undergo hot water washing, which is the way everything is washed in the nursing home.

Some days are just bad days. The day after her birthday, Sara was at the door when I arrived. Her first words were, "Are we going home today?" It's the first time she has actually said it like that. I told her, "This is your home now." She didn't say anything after that. It turned out to be a depressing day for me.

On December 12, I met Mr. Gallup at the county social services office to submit Sara's Medi-Cal application. The application and supporting documentation was one hundred and thirty two pages long. It covered personal, medical, social and educational, work history and three years of financial records covering every aspect of assets and income for both Sara and myself.

The social services case worker apparently had handled a lot of Medi-Cal cases, because she went through the paperwork like clockwork, asking an occasional question, making notations, taking notes and highlighting items. Mr. Gallup, didn't have much to say during the interview, because I had done everything just like he told me, and thus there were few questions to be asked by the caseworker.

At the conclusion of the application interview, I was told, "You will hear the results of the application within forty-five days." Mr. Gallup said, "Let me know as soon as you receive the results of the application." I told him I would.

Over the next few days, every time I arrived to visit Sara, she would be at the door waiting. The staff says she spends much of her time just standing at the door waiting for me. It really bothers me that she is doing this.

> The operation apparently did the job, because Sara's chronic trips to the bathroom have finally stopped. It had to have been a miserable time for her over the months, unable to tell anyone exactly what her problem was.

Spud has been having problems. She can't get up and down the steps at home and hasn't been eating. On December 18, when I tried to get Spud up to drink some water, she just fell over. I took Spud to the vet, who announced, "She's suffering from congestive heart failure." The vet saw no favorable prognosis and thus I had Spud put to sleep. I took Spud home from the vet and buried her next to Lucy. Now I was totally alone, except for Spot.

The next day, I told Sara that Spud died. She had no response. I would keep telling her each time she asked how Spud was doing over the weeks ahead and each time she would look surprised.

Darby flew down from Portland on December 21. After picking her up at the San Diego airport, we stopped off to see Sara. They were having an early Christmas party with Santa Claus and crew. There was a big crowd. Sara got two presents from Santa Claus. She was quite happy and did a few Hokey Pokey's for us.

Amy, Marc and Kyle and their two dogs arrived home two days before Christmas. Kyle immediately became ill, which did not make for a good holiday season.

I had contemplated bringing Sara home, but decided against it, again. We all went down and visited Sara on Christmas day. We took presents, but she couldn't open them by herself. What she got were new clothes and she didn't seem to act very excited about them. There was a time when new clothes would have had her dancing around, trying everything on, but no longer.

Christmas got worse as Darby and Marc joined Kyle in becoming ill.

The day after Christmas, the nursing home reported, "Sara has broken out in a rash. We called Dr. Newhous for directions as to how to treat it"

My 61st birthday, December 27, saw Darby still very ill. The rest of us took Sara out to lunch at the Boll Weevil and then for a drive along the coast. Sara held Kyle and really seemed to enjoy his company.

I received notice that Sara's care was going to be increased from $96 to $99 per day for her semi-private room. I let the director of the Alzheimer's section know that I had submitted an application for Medi-Cal for Sara and I was just waiting for the results.

I took Darby to the airport on December 29. On the way, we stopped off and visited Sara. Sara seemed fine except for her body rash, which they were treating when we arrived.

Chapter 21

I Love You,
You Are Special

*T*he year 1996 began with my meeting with the director of the nursing home to discuss Sara's application for Medi-Cal. Although the nursing home accepted Medi-Cal patients, they said they had a waiting list for Medi-Cal patients whose coverage was for semi-private rooms only. Sara had been admitted as a private patient into a private room. After two months though, she was moved to a semi-private room. The director saw no problem with Sara qualifying for Medi-Cal at this time.

For the next couple of weeks I took Sara for rides to discover places I was not familiar with, as well as to the beach, where we would watch the surfers. We had lunch together a few times. Since I no longer spent day and night caring for Sara's physical concerns, we actually got to enjoy each other the most that could be expected in a situation like ours

Every day Sara would ask, "How's Spud?" and each time I would tell her, "Spud has died." She always looks surprised when I tell her, as if she had never asked the question or heard my reply.

Sara's standing and waiting by the main entrance for hours had apparently caused problems for staff members so they said to me, "Can you start coming to a side entrance to the Alzheimer's wing of the nursing home? There is a bench there, where Sara can sit and wait for you." I agreed. The idea was to try to get Sara used to me coming through a different door.

On each visit Sara keeps saying, "I love you," and, "You are special." I guess I should be happy when she says it, but it actually makes me sad. Sometimes I think Sara has the advantage of being only in the present. I remember the past only too painfully and am so aware of our future. No wonder I feel sad much of the time.

I received, by mail, on January 26, a "Notice of Action," from the Department of Social Services, Health and Welfare Agency, State of California telling me that Sara qualified for Medicaid/Medi-Cal effective on February 1st. I called Mr. Gallup to let him know and to thank him. As far as I was concerned he had certainly earned his $1000. The nursing home received similar notification. That was certainly a weight off of my mind.

The process was finally completed, nearly a year after I started it. During the past year I had spent over $34,000 on Sara's medical care. I guess all I can do is be grateful that through our hard work we had the $34,000 to spend on her care. Of course, it would have been much better if we had known to buy long-term care insurance. Even though the statistics quoted are that 45% of people in long-term care situations are under age 65, we had no awareness of long-term care insurance before we needed it, and it's like fire insurance, you can't get it when your house burns down, you need it before.

On occasion I would bring some birdseed with me and have Sara feed the sea gulls and pigeons at the beach where we visited. At first she was still cognizant enough to enjoy feeding them, but as time passed, she seemed to enjoy it less and less. I was sad to see another activity that we enjoyed together, disappear from our lives.

When Valentine's Day arrived, the nursing home sponsored a Valentine's Ball. Everyone was dressed up. The home provided Sara with an evening gown that actually fit her. Her weight was up to 146 pounds. When I asked her, "How much do you weigh?" the answer is always "110."

We danced a few times, even today she was still my sweetheart. We had a good time together.

February 23 was the first anniversary of Sara being in the nursing home. We took a drive to the beach. Sara said, "I love you." I told her, "I love you too." I asked her, "Will you marry me?" She said, "No." I said nothing in response.

The nursing home changed ownership in February. Changes in

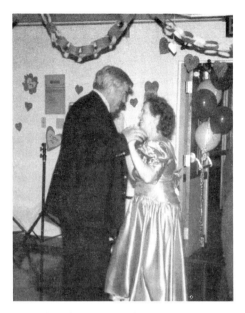

personnel happened almost immediately. A lot of the employees I thought were very positive assets to the nursing home, started disappearing and were replaced with new faces and names to learn. I talked to the head of the Alzheimer's unit when she announced she was leaving. She let me know that the new policies being introduced were not part of her philosophy, and she was leaving for other employment. I could only hope this would not adversely affect Sara.

Amy, Marc and Kyle came down for Easter. Sara could not place Kyle. He was just a "little boy." After a while of holding him, she finally seemed to have some feeling for him. She always loved little babies. On April 13, Corbin and I picked up Sara and drove for two hours to Long Beach to visit Amy and family. She just sat and looked at Kyle, saying nothing. Then we drove back another two hours. It was our longest time out together in a long time. She did well.

Our 34th wedding anniversary was April 14. There was not much to celebrate and I felt really depressed. I took Sara to lunch and we visited the beach.

Then I took a trip to Oregon for a week where it rained everyday. When I got back and went to visit Sara, she didn't indicate that I had even been gone. She again said, "You are special," and, "I love you." I showed her pictures of my trip to Oregon. She did not recognize my mother, Darby or Darby's dog "Bela." When I told her the dog's name was Bela, she recognized our oldest daughter, Darby. She did recognize her mother's picture.

May was a busy month. Corbin and I often visited Sara together. On visiting, I would usually have to hunt for Sara and it was not unusual to find her in someone else's room lying on a bed.

It was time for the quarterly meeting with the nursing home employees about Sara's care. My registered concern was Sara's weight gain. They indicated that it is difficult to control Sara's eating because she would take food from the plates of other patients.

Almost all of Sara's clothes, I still had at home, were no longer suitable for her to wear, either because of her weight gain, or their style, so I donated them to the local Alzheimer's Thrift Store. Now she just wears simple clothing like long pants, shirts and sweaters. She wears no jewelry or make up, but she does seem to enjoy having her fingernails painted.

We continued our rides to the beach and occasional meals out during the summer. For whatever reason, Sara stopped doing the Hokey Pokey and asking about Spud. I would continue to find Sara asleep in a chair or in a room on someone else's bed.

As a rule, Sara does not talk, but will respond with minimum words when asked a question. One day she actually tried to talk and tell me something, but could not complete her thoughts and finally just stopped and became silent. On a couple of other occasions Sara would try to say a sentence, but would never be able to complete it.

I would often find Sara in the original room she had when she first entered the nursing home. She seems to think that it is still her room, although it has been over a year since she resided there.

In late August I met with the nursing staff to go over Sara's quarterly care plan. I was not particularly impressed with the presentation. Seems like every quarter, when going over the plan, it's always with a new bunch of employees. I have noticed that there is a large, and consistent, turnover in the nursing home employees. I'm not quite sure what the problem is, whether it's the working conditions at the home or the low pay. My real concern was Sara's care, and that did not seem to be affected. The new people took care of Sara as well as the people who had left.

In early September, I went to Oregon to see my mother and sister in Corvallis and Darby in Portland. On returning, I found Sara waiting at the door. It's as if I had not been gone at all. She said she loved me and that I was special. I don't know why, but it makes me feel depressed.

Our drives to the beach are much nicer now that the summer crowds are gone. The surfers are still present, but not in the same numbers.

The nursing home finally installed locks on the closets in the patient's rooms, in an attempt to get better control of the clothing situation.

> Every time I bring new clothes for Sara, they get logged into her file, for what reason I do not know, it sure doesn't keep them from disappearing. One day on checking Sara's shoe supply I found five unmatched shoes. Although I always put on name labels or write her name on the clothing when I bring clothing items, they seem to disappear after awhile. Maybe the locks will change that now.

In some cases, I find Sara in clothes that no longer fit or are functional, that is, with elastic bands that no longer keep her trousers up. I throw away the old item so no one will try to dress her in it again.

In October, during a remodeling project, the carpet was removed from the patient's rooms and replaced with vinyl flooring. The staff says it was much easier to clean the rooms without the carpeting. I must say, that for the most part, the cleaning staff does a very good job of keeping the nursing home clean. Seldom are there any offensive odors.

I am starting to notice the occasional disappearance of patients. You see the same faces day after day, then you realize that so and so is no longer around, and you have not seen them for some time. On a couple of occasions I have asked the staff what happen to so and so and the generic response is, "I don't know." I can only surmise it is policy not to discuss patients that disappear for any reason, i.e., moved out of the Alzheimer's wing, or moved into the skilled nursing wing, or died.

The doors to the Alzheimer's wing of the nursing home have two little windows that look down the corridor everyone must use to enter the locked wing. That is where Sara, along with other patients, would stand and look out literally for hours on end. It was often a hindrance for the staff moving in and out of the locked facility. Finally someone got the idea to mask the windows, so patients could not just stand there and stare down the corridor. It seemed to work, because I would find Sara less and less around the entry doors.

In October 1996, Sara got a letter to renew her driver's license. I sent the notification back with a note and her driver's license, indicating that she had Alzheimer's disease and was no longer driving. In early November I got a letter from DMV suspending her driving privileges. The last time Sara had driven a car was May 27, 1994 at which time I had taken her car keys away and become her chauffeur.

As required by law, Dr. Newhous would visit Sara monthly to examine her physical condition. I happened to see him only once when he was visiting Sara and his other patients in the nursing home. According to the nurses, more often than not, Dr. Newhous' visits were in the late evening, often quite late and never announced. Certainly this didn't please me. He may have complied with the law in this manner, but unless he came on a night that Sara was up, which was not consistent, then he could only go over her records, or wake her up to examine her.

Periodically, I would take Sara to see Dr. Smith to check her medication. Sara no longer recognizes Dr. Smith, after nearly four years of visits to him.

Sara is becoming more and more quiet. She often greets me with, "I love you," and then says not another word. No longer do I hear her say, "You're special," which used to accompany, "I love you." Even when I try to get her to say something, she usually cannot respond. She does not know how old she is or how much she weighs. She has difficulty remembering the children's names and on some days cannot remember at all. She can no longer remember her only grandson, Kyle, and was never able to associate who he really was.

Corbin, Amy and family, and a friend were home for Thanksgiving. It was a quiet event and with Sara's condition, it was difficult for any of us to feel thankful.

December 1, Sara and I went to Solana Beach and watched another surfing contest. On returning to the nursing home, we rang the doorbell to gain entrance to the Alzheimer's wing. As we waited for someone to open the door, I heard the sound of water. I looked, and Sara was wetting her pants as we stood there. She seemed oblivious to what was happening. According to the nurses this was the first time she had done this. Sara always told me when she had to go to the bathroom, but not this time. I was hoping that this was just an "accident," but afraid it is the just the beginning of full incontinence.

December 9 was Sara's 61st birthday. I told her, "It's December 9th. Does that date mean anything to you?" She said, "It's my birthday." This really surprised me and I smiled. Then I asked, "How old are you today?" She said, "Pretty old." I told her, "You are sixty-one now." There was no reply, just a vacant stare.

Procedural progress was made on December 12!

It was always the procedure that guests visiting the Alzheimer's wing of the nursing home had to ring a doorbell to gain entrance. This required some waiting, until one of the nurse's aides could come to the door, enter the secret code, known only to the employees, and let the guest in. Today, the code was posted at the entrance, so now guests could let themselves in without waiting. The initial catch was you had to remember the code to get out, because it was not posted inside the wing. This was a big time saver for all involved, particularly the employees who had to stop whatever they were doing to let guests in and out. I liked some of the changes with the new administration, more control of clothing, vinyl floors for easier cleaning, and now the code for more ease in entering and leaving the Alzheimer's wing.

The nursing home had a Christmas party on December 19. Compared to last year it was poorly organized, with not nearly enough seating available. Carolers were present to sing songs. Sara sang along with "Jingle Bells," and seemed to get every word right. It made me happy and proud of her. I was beginning to understand more and more that although she couldn't formulate new words or create recent memories, she could still access her long-term memory with coaching, especially through music.

On Christmas, Amy, Marc, Kyle, Corbin and I visited Sara and took presents to her. It was depressing when Sara could not manage to open her gifts. Her concentration didn't seem to last long enough to open a gift, nor did she have the physical dexterity to open them. Of course, we helped her. Sara's emotional response had decreased to the point that she did not act excited about anything she received.

To celebrate the end of 1996 on New Year's Eve, I went to the nursing home to take Sara for a ride. When I arrived, I found her asleep in a chair. I just sat with her until she woke up. Then I took her for a ride to the beach while we watched the waves together in silence. Once she gave me one of her smiles, which still captivated me after all these years.

Chapter 22

Are You Taking
Me Home?

*T*he New Year 1997 started off cold and rainy and I was called for jury duty. I was named twice to serve on two juries, but each time I was challenged off, apparently because I had known the judge for nearly forty years.

On January 11, I picked Darby up at the San Diego airport. We stopped and visited Sara. We found her asleep in a chair. She recognized Darby, which pleased us. She was mostly silent though.

Early February, I got Sara a Valentine's card to send to her mother. With great effort, I got her to write, "I love you, Sara." Her writing was so small and it was a real struggle for her, but she managed. I knew the card would mean so much to Grammy who was now having a great deal of difficulty with her physical body as well.

A meeting was announced to discuss the care being given to the patients. The nursing home had acquired new leadership again and it was to be sort of an orientation, and give and take meeting. Six spouses showed up for the meeting. Various issues were discussed. I provided a two page letter of some of my concerns and/or observations. Everyone got to speak their mind on various subjects, which proved beneficial to all concerned.

Sara and I continued to take rides to the beach and made an occasional visit to the Boll Weevil. The nursing home employees continued to have problems getting Sara properly dressed, including getting her to wear a bra. She has all the clothes she needs, but getting them on her sometimes seems to be a challenge. Sara can no longer dress herself.

She went through a period of an upper respiratory problem causing her to suffer severe coughing spells. It took a couple of weeks for her to get over that. Chest x-rays ruled out pneumonia.

March 17, I received a phone call from the nursing home at 6:30 p.m. It was a very distressing call! The nurse said, "Sara has been molested by another patient. A nursing aid heard Sara making noises and saw a male patient with one hand on her crotch and one on her breast. The nursing aid immediately stopped it. Sara was not physically injured. Everything is under control now." The nurse further said, "I've called Dr. Newhous, Sara's doctor, who also happens to be the doctor for the male patient. You can call Dr. Newhous." It was apparent that there was nothing I could do, they were taking care of the situation to the best of their ability. Still it unnerved me.

The next morning, I went to the nursing home and started investigating the molestation. The director of the Alzheimer's unit, Mr. Carren, indicated that if everything goes well, the offending male patient would be out of the facility by nightfall. The nursing home leadership would not tell me who the male patient was, but I had my suspicions.

Mr. Carren told me, "The male patient has had his medication increased so as to provide further medical restraint on his actions. He has been placed on a fifteen minute watch, which means his location and actions will be checked every fifteen minutes. Also, all the employees have been made aware of the situation and are to be more watchful over Sara." Mr. Carren also informed me, "Sara is not the only victim, the male patient accosted another female patient a few days ago."

After my discussion with the director of the Alzheimer's unit and the nurses, I went looking for Sara. I found her asleep in a chair. The first thing she said to me was, "Are you taking me home?" It was the first time she has mentioned "home" in a long time. I was saddened by the question and really didn't know what to say, so I just said nothing.

On each visit, I would ask, "Is the male patient who accosted Sara still around?" Finally Mr. Carren told me, "It turns out we can not evict him from the home, his family does not want to move him." Although it may be difficult to get someone into a nursing home, once there, it is apparently nearly impossible to get them out. Apparently there are laws which provide protection to patients and in this case, they could not evict him. They assured me however, he was being watched, as was Sara.

The nursing home had a beauty parlor in the Alzheimer's wing, which the entire nursing home used. I had been taking Sara to her old hairdresser in Vista, but it was getting difficult for the hairdresser to control her, so I decided to use the one in the nursing home. The operator, Linda Dixon, only worked two mornings a week, but was very busy. Linda didn't work directly for the nursing home, but I would be billed by the nursing home, which in turn would pay her. Although she did not work for the nursing home, she could have been one of their top employees the way she cared for the patients. One day she told me that she started at the nursing home by cutting her father's hair, who was a patient there. After he died, she continued to take care of the patients. Linda was, and still is, a tremendous asset to the home.

On March 25, I had to sign a form called, "Authorization or Withdraw Life-Sustaining/Life-Prolonging Measures." I provided the nursing home a copy of Sara's "Durable Power of Attorney - For Health Care," which Sara had signed May 11, 1992, just prior to her problems really surfacing. At the time she signed it, she indicated, ". . .being of sound mind, I willingly and voluntarily make known my desire that my life shall not be artificially prolonged. . ." We had both signed our durable power of attorney documents on the same day, both with the same statement included.

A few months later, she could not have signed such a document stating "being of sound mind."

After some thought on the matter, I decided that I should obtain long-term care insurance for myself. I could see that if you did not have the insurance in place while you could still qualify, then you would never be able to obtain it when you needed it.

With Sara "gone," I was on my own, as I saw it. I did not want to burden my children with my care, should I ever need it. Of course the statistics indicated that I just might need it sometime in my life. I checked around and referred back to some of the seminar material I had accumulated on the subject. As a retired teacher in California, I was qualified to apply for long-term care through the California public employee's (CalPERS) organization. In April, I applied for long-term care insurance through CalPERS. In July 1997, I was informed I had been accepted and my coverage would commence starting August 1. My monthly premium was set at $112 per month for the type of coverage I had applied for.

Sara is becoming quieter. She only said things such as, "What did you do today?" and "You have big shoes," or "Your hair looks good," . . . just little sentences and then nothing after that. I often asked Sara questions like, "How old are you? How long have we been married? How much do you weigh? What are the names of our children?" She can no longer answer the questions.

April 9, Donna and Roger Ryman visited Sara. They were in San Diego from Colorado for a business meeting and had called ahead to arrange to see Sara. Donna was Sara's sorority sister at Oregon State. We had been friends for a long time, I had recruited Roger into the Marine Corps back in 1958 while he was a student at Oregon State. I was pleased they made arrangements to visit. So often we hear about people with illnesses not being visited by their old friends–they no longer have things in common with each other and see no reason to continue to visit a person who receives them without enthusiasm.

On April 11, I got another call from the nursing home reporting, "Sara has been molested again. It is the same man." I told the nurse that I was on my way to the nursing home and I wanted to see the director of the Alzheimer's unit when I got there.

On arriving, the director was waiting for me. He was somewhat defensive. He said, "I'm sorry, but it's nearly impossible to evict the male patient. Sara approaches the man apparently because she might think he resembles you. We are trying to keep them separated and both are continually being watched by the staff." It was not a good day.

Eventually the man I suspected, just disappeared. But that was not unusual, because patients were always disappearing from the nursing home and where they went, I would never know, except in one instance I knew because a patient had unexpectedly died just as I arrived at the home one day, which had the staff hustling around.

On my visits I would bring Sara orange juice and I would have coffee. We would either go for a ride, sit on the patio or sit out front of the nursing home.

Sara could still speak, but would say little. She would say some things that were kind of funny. Things like:

- ♦   You sure are a big boy.
- ♦   The traffic is really loud.
- ♦   Your hair looks nice.
- ♦   You sure are handsome.
- ♦   Your eyebrows have gray hair in them.
- ♦   You sure have a red face.

There was no conversation she just made statements, followed by silence.

One day I told her I was sixty-two years old. I asked her, "How old are you?" She said, "Thirty-six." I'm not sure how she came up with that number.

When Sara first entered the home, all the patients had wrist bracelets for identification, but so many of the patients would play with them and twist them and eventually they would break off. So now they moved the identification bracelets to the ankles. The only problem was that often I would find Sara's ankle bracelet forced up her leg which would affect her circulation and she would not even know it.

One day I received a letter and photographs from one of Sara's sorority sisters. Sara's sorority class of 1958 had a reunion of which Sara was the only one absent. I showed the pictures to Sara and she could not name a single woman in her class. I pointed out several that I remembered and told her their names. On occasion she would smile when I mentioned a name, but never said a word.

In May, Sara developed eating problems. She would not pick up a fork or spoon, but would just sit in front of her plate. On occasion I would try and help her eat. Finally the staff put her into a special program, where they would try to teach her to eat all over again. There were three or four others undergoing the same retraining.

When going for rides in the car, Sara could still fasten her seat belt automatically, but she could not unfasten it. She could still apply lipstick by herself, which I brought with me. I guess that, just out of habit, she could physically do little routine things.

It was in the summer of 1997 that Sara started developing a rocking motion. She would just sit and rock from side to side. She was very quiet and said little, even when coaxed and encouraged.

I continued to note continual changes on visiting Sara. She used to wait by the door a lot, but not anymore. It used to be that when I came to visit and would find her, she would noticed me and come to see me. Now, if she is sitting somewhere and sees me, she doesn't get up, she just rocks back and forth and looks at me. The rocking is increasing.

I had been having a lot of problems with my left foot, I get a callus buildup that causes a lot of pain in walking. So every few weeks I needed to see a podiatrist to cut the callus off. On a couple of occasions I had gotten infections that required laceration and draining. This had been going on for some time and the podiatrist said, "The only possible solution would be an operation, but that would put you off your feet for eight to ten weeks. Plus, there is no guarantee the operation would cure the problem."

After nearly a month of going through the retraining program for eating, they took Sara off the program. She was not progressing.

The duty nurse said the staff would help her eat, like they do with several other patients. Fortunately, after several weeks, for no reason, Sara started feeding herself again. Depending upon what was being served, the staff would have to cut up her food, but she could handle either fork or spoon. She had no trouble handling burgers, which she still enjoys.

When I visited Sara now, after only a few minutes she would often just get up and walk away from me. I tried to get her to say something on every visit, but seldom did she say anything. She would still smile when someone called her name.

I continued to take Sara to our dentist for checkups and cleaning. Her teeth are really not what they use to be. She generally did a good job at the dentist office, although she tried on occasion to get out of the chair. The dentist and hygienist were very patient with Sara, who on occasion can be a little difficult.

August 12, I flew to Portland, Oregon to visit with Darby, and Don and Pat, my brother and sister in law. I took a trip to Corvallis to see my mother and sister, Virginia. At age 84, my mother finally moved into a retirement home. I told my mother, "If and when you move into a retirement home, I will be one of your first visitors," which I was. It was a very nice facility, but mother did not really enjoy it. She had taken most of the family pictures she had collected over the years to decorate the walls of her room, but she was really not happy. She could not take care of herself any longer in her own home, thus the move was absolutely necessary.

My first visit to Sara upon returning home found her sitting in the recreation room in her favorite spot, which was a corner couch near a window. When she saw me, she didn't seem to recognize who I was. Sometimes I feel she does not know me any longer. I am just a guy that brings her orange juice and takes her for a ride. I got her to say my name, as well as her own, one time, but there was no recognition in the words. She was just repeating what I said.

After visiting Sara on August 26, when I arrived home I had a message to call the nursing home. I had not seen the nurse on my visit that day. The nurse informed me that one of the male patients had hit Sara in the head five or six times the night before. Sara had been sitting in a chair that the male patient wanted to use to watch

TV. He had hit other patients before. The nurse explained, "For some reason the man feels that certain chairs are his and often when he wants to use them anyone sitting in them is accosted." The nurse further informed me, "We got a private TV to put in the man's room, which we hope will resolve the problem." When visiting Sara that day I had looked carefully, but saw no evidence that she had been hit on her face or head. The nurse reassured me saying, "We didn't find any injury to Sara's head."

> It's times like this, that I really get depressed. I know the nursing home staff is doing their best, but when you have so many Alzheimer's patients grouped together, each in various stages of the disease, it's obvious that problems will develop. On more than one occasion I have seen the patients become hostile with both the employees and other patients.

The first week in September, I noticed that the gold identification bracelet, which I had gotten Sara, was missing. The bracelet was part of the "Safe Return" program that I had enrolled Sara in a couple of years earlier. I reported the bracelet missing. The bracelet is of the type that takes two hands to fasten or unfasten, so I knew Sara could not have taken it off herself. Later I took a picture of what the bracelet looked liked, so everyone would know what to look for. The bracelet never turned up, so after a couple of weeks I ordered another one.

On September 4, I found Sara in the recreation room. I took her outside to the patio and in doing so found that she had wet her pants and was soaking wet and totally oblivious to it. I took her to the nurse, who had Sara changed. I discussed the situation with the nurse. She said, "This is happening more often now. We're trying to get her to go to bathroom more frequently."

I attended my Marine Corps 3-57 officers basic class reunion held in San Diego the weekend of September 13. It was a pretty good turnout with many old friends in attendance. Another event Sara missed.

One day Sara and I were sitting out front of the nursing home having our coffee and orange juice. We were just watching the traffic go by on the freeway and as trucks went by, I asked Sara what the name was on one of the trucks. She said, "Lucky." She was right. Of course she always shopped at our local Lucky store in Vista, so was familiar the logo.

On other days while we sat out front, I started asking her to name trucks, color of trucks and whatever else I thought would get her to say something. She got all kinds of trucks right: Pepsi, Vons, Ralphs, Albertsons, 7-Up, U-Haul, Mayflower, Circuit City, Bekins, Ryder, school bus, Wal-Mart and Lucky. Every once in awhile she would miss the name on a truck, but seldom missed on Lucky trucks. She could also tell me the colors of trucks I pointed to: "red" trucks, "yellow" trucks, "white" trucks, etc. She usually smiled and looked happy when she named a truck.

Sara turned sixty-two on December 9, 1997. Mr. Gallup, my Medi-Cal consultant had informed me that anytime Sara was entitled to a benefit, she must apply for it. So, in this case, at age sixty-two, Sara was eligible for Social Security benefits, based on my earnings. So I applied to Social Security for benefits in her name. She would not receive much, only around $300 a month. Of that, all but $35 per month would be paid to the nursing home to offset the cost of her care. Commencing January 1998, Sara started receiving benefits. I informed the nursing home of this, so they could bill me appropriately.

I never had the courage to take Sara back home since she had been in the nursing home. Last Christmas the children and I discussed bring Sara home for Christmas day, but finally decided against it.

This year, I decided that bringing Sara home for Christmas day would not cause her any difficulty.

Amy, Marc, Kyle and Corbin were home for Christmas. I went to the nursing home Christmas morning to pick Sara up and bring her back home. On the drive home Sara said nothing and hardly even looked around. In Vista, we passed the middle school our children had attended. I asked her what the name of the school was. She said, "Lincoln." She was right, but that is all she said. As we passed the local park where she used to play tennis every day, I asked her the name of the park and she said, "Brengle." She was right again. Those would be the only two words she would say all day.

I was not sure what to expect at home and I knew I had to keep an eye on her all day. She walked around the house very little. Mostly she just sat in the living room, watching and listening to Christmas music.

She paid little attention to opening her Christmas presents, I had to help her. Although I tried to get her to the bathroom on a regular basis throughout the day, she still wet her pants once. Clean up was necessary.

Sara smiled a lot and rocked to the Christmas music. We had a nice dinner and Sara did a good job of eating. She seemed to have an enjoyable day.

The ride back to the nursing home was uneventful. By bedtime I was exhausted. It had been a very stressful day for me, but I was glad that I had brought Sara home to be with us, even though she was no longer the mother, but the child.

Chapter 23

She Cares for Me

*W*e started off the New Year of 1998 sitting in front of the nursing home having our usual coffee and orange juice. Sara can still name a few trucks, which surprises me and makes me happy.

I got her to say "Vern," and better yet, I got her to spell, "S-A-R-A." Each day is becoming different. Some days I can get her to say a word or two and other days, not a sound.

On January 16, I took Sara to the dentist. He said her teeth are in great shape. I sure hope they stay that way.

Over the holidays I finally made the decision to undergo a foot operation. The operation would entail cutting the bone of my little toe on my left foot, realigning it and putting a pin in it.

I had to do some planning in preparation for the operation. I would be off my feet for nearly three months and would have to use crutches and a wheelchair. It was necessary that I rearrange my house for handling a wheelchair. I also saw a need to hire the neighbor's son to do odd jobs for me. Don and Pat were again wintering in Oceanside, and Don took me for the surgery on January

24 and then picked me up later and took me home. I could drive fine, because it was my left foot that underwent the surgery. I would crutch my way to the car and take off.

Visiting Sara turned out to be a real hassle. Depending on the parking situation at the nursing home, it could be a ways to get inside the home. It was also a long hall to get to Sara's location and then I'd have to walk even more to find her. On my first visit it took some time to find Sara. I could not hold onto her and still use the crutches, so I ended up just sitting and watching Sara walk the halls.

On my next visit, the nursing home let me borrow a wheelchair, which made a world of difference. I rolled along trying to keep up with Sara as she walked the halls. Then one of the attendants said, "Why don't you have Sara push you in the wheelchair? Sara often pushes other patients around." He got her behind the wheelchair and off we went! She pushed me all over the place, in and out of foot and wheelchair traffic. She did a great job! We didn't hit anyone or anything. I guess she finally got tired of it all and just walked off.

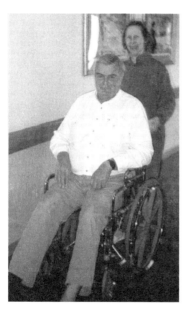

One day I had to take Sara to see Dr. Smith for a medication check. I couldn't do it by myself on crutches, so I got my brother Don to go with me. If someone doesn't hang onto Sara, she will just walk away.

February 7, marked the first day that Sara wore diapers during the day. The staff had been putting diapers on her at night for some time, but now diapers were to be fulltime, she had finally reached the stage of complete incontinence.

Sara was going through another bout with an upper respiratory infection. She was constantly coughing and very tired all the time.

Sara still pushed me in the wheelchair, but would often just stop and walk off. At least I could follow her around in the wheelchair, or just sit and wait for her to reappear.

One day I took some pictures for Sara to look at. She was able to name Corbin, Kyle, herself and me. Some days she knows and other days she does not.

On March 4, I managed to load my wheelchair into my car and headed for Long Beach. Today Amy was to deliver our second grandchild by cesarean birth. The sex of the child was not determined before birth as was the case with Kyle. Amy and Marc wanted to be surprised. Finally Ethan Sheldon Prager was delivered, weighing in at 9 pounds, 14 ounces.

The following day I informed Sara, "You're a grandmother again." As expected it meant nothing to her. It would have meant a great deal to her when she was well, but she wasn't.

Her continued coughing had gotten to the point that Dr. Newhous ordered a "barium swallow" performed. The problem was, I had to get her to the hospital to do it, and on crutches I needed help, so I recruited an old Marine Corps friend of forty years, for assistance. I delivered Sara to the hospital for the procedure. However, her condition was such that the doctor asked me to assist. So, while sitting on a chair, I helped station Sara before the x-ray equipment as she swallowed the barium solution. It was a difficult procedure, but somehow Sara got it done. The test results turned out negative.

Dr. Newhous had no solution for Sara's coughing. Eventually Sara just recovered.

My visits with Sara were just about all the same now. She might push me around in a wheelchair, but eventually she would just walk off. There was little I could do about it.

On the weekend of March 22, Darby and her fiancé flew down from Portland. They were here for just the weekend and were busy moving around visiting. They went to Long Beach to see Amy and family. We visited Sara and were able to sit out in front of the nursing home. Sara named one U-Haul truck and was able to say Darby's name, which made Darby happy.

The foot surgeon removed the pin from my foot on April 4 and said I could walk a little.

> Finally after nearly ten weeks I was liberated from the crutches and the wheelchair! Now I was able to take Sara orange juice and we could go for rides again!

On April 5, Amy, Marc, Kyle and Ethan came to visit Sara. It was the first time that Sara had seen Ethan. She held Ethan and seemed to enjoy him. Kyle still wouldn't let Sara hold him. Kyle played ball with Sara, bouncing a big rubber ball back and forth. Sara was very good at bouncing the ball, it is one of the activities that she enjoys participating in at the nursing home during their exercise periods.

The nursing home provides several different types of exercises, from stretching to bouncing balls, to rhythmic exercises with music. The following day I took Sara to see Dr. Smith. He decided to take her off her medication, which was Zoloft. He wanted to see her in a couple of months or sooner, if there were any significant changes.

I met with the nursing home staff to go over Sara's quarterly care plan. This particular meeting was not very well prepared and the information on her medication was incorrect—she was no longer taking Zoloft.

I took Sara out for her first ride, other than to see Dr. Smith, in three months. We went to the beach as we usually did and had our coffee and orange juice. Sara rocked to the music on the radio. She still keeps pretty good time to the beat of the music. I enjoyed my time with Sara.

I reminded Sara on April 14, "It's our thirty-fifth wedding anniversary." No reaction.

As May moved along, I took Sara on rides, or we just sat out in front of the nursing home. Some days she could name trucks, some days not. Of course I liked it when she named a truck, but even more I just liked being with my Sara. Her presence is still there.

Besides the rocking motion Sara had developed, she was now in the habit of slapping her legs and clapping her hands. It seemed to be just a spontaneous impulse for her to do these things.

A visit to the dentist in June was a little difficult. Sara slapped her legs while in the dentist chair, which caused some disruption. The dentist said her gums were not in very good shape. He wrote a note to the nursing home indicating a need for better dental hygiene. Her gums are tender and often bleed when her teeth are brushed. The nurses already assist Sara with brushing her teeth twice daily. They also give her an oral rinse after brushing, and it's on her chart to observe gums for any bleeding, redness, tenderness and break down. Even with that much assistance, her gums continued to deteriorate.

When I got home one day, I had a message on my answering service from the nursing home. Apparently Sara had been hitting herself hard rather frequently and it was suggested that I make an appointment to have Dr. Smith, the psychiatrist, see her, which I did. The nursing staff encouraged Sara to attend activities, to help relieve some of the agitation. They would gently hold her hands a moment when she slapped herself to get her to stop.

> Today when I visited Sara she came right to me when she saw me and I even managed to get a hug from her. We sat out front and had our coffee and orange juice. Today Sara could not name a truck, or say even one word.

We visited Dr. Smith and he prescribed medication for Sara that he felt might help her overcome the agitation she seemed to be feeling. It was a difficult visitation, Sara kept trying to get away, causing me to actually have to restrain her, which was something I didn't like doing.

Over the next couple of weeks, the medication prescribed by Dr. Smith seemed to have some beneficial effect in controlling Sara's slapping and clapping, which could be rather harsh at times. One day I got her to say, "Vern," "Sara," and "Darby." It became routine that I had to hunt for Sara when I visited the nursing home. She didn't walk around as much as she used to, and seldom is she ever by the entrance door anymore. She had a favorite spot in the dining/recreation room—a couch in the corner by a window. Sometimes I would find her lying on a bed, either awake or a sleep.

Her slapping and clapping continues, and, on occasion, she will even slap my leg as we are sitting together, but that is seldom.

Another visit to Dr. Smith resulted in a small increase in her medication. The nurses think the medication seemed to have some slight affect.

On visiting Sara a few days later, after another fishing trip which gave me a break and a chance to visit with friends, I found her lying on a bed, as usual not in her own room. When she saw me, she got up and came to me. We took a ride to the beach and had our coffee and orange juice. She gently slapped her legs.

A couple of days later we were sitting out front, Sara was coughing and then she suddenly vomited. I took her to the nurse who said she would monitor Sara.

Sara was still doing well with naming trucks, as we would sit in front of the nursing home.

In September, on one of our visits, Amy, Marc, Kyle and Ethan and myself were sitting on the patio. There were some tomato plants growing in a planter on the patio. I asked Sara, "What are these plants?" and she replied, "I don't know." It was the first time she had said more then a single word in a long time. I got Sara to say Amy's name, which pleased all of us. Sara and Kyle played catch with one of the big balls they used for exercise times at the nursing home. Kyle gave Sara three big hugs. It was the first time he would let Sara get close enough to hug him since he was a baby.

We continued to take rides to the beach or sit out front. She would clap her hands or slap her legs, but the frequency and severity changed from day to day. Some days Sara seemed happy and other days, sad or tired. I was beginning to notice her feelings more and more.

In late September, Sara was frequently looking tired and seemed congested. The doctor prescribed medication for her.

On October 3, at 1:30 a.m., I got a call from the nursing home. Sara apparently had a reaction to the medication and the duty nurse was going to have her transported to the hospital. I got up and drove to the nursing home. When I arrived, they had decided not to send her to the hospital, but to monitor her condition closely. Her blood pressure was 102/64 and had been somewhat lower earlier. Sara had broken out in a rash. She was sleeping.

The next day I found her asleep in her own bed, for once. When she woke up, I gave her orange juice and it was apparent she was very thirsty. She looked a lot better, but still had a body rash. Her pulse was 84. It had been over a 100 when she suffered her reaction to the medication. She was in good spirits and I got her to say, "Vern," "Sara," and "toe."

The next few days, she seemed tired, but was getting better. She could still name the trucks, although she would miss some. When I say miss some, I mean she would say nothing when I asked her to name a truck.

I told Sara, "I'm going to fly to Oregon on October 14th to attend Darby's wedding." Darby, at age 33, was getting married. Sara had no idea what I was talking about. Sara was to miss another event that would have meant so much to her.

When I came back on Tuesday, I told her about the wedding, but I was really just talking to myself. Even the mention of Darby's name didn't seem to mean anything to her.

A trip to the dentist had Sara's teeth and gums looking a little better over the last visit. But x-rays revealed a need for a filling.

Sara is not walking as much as she used to. I usually just find her lying on a bed somewhere. Over the years, she has undoubtedly been on all sixty beds in the Alzheimer's wing. After only a few minutes of being with her, she will often just get up and walk away. I can't restrain her because she will forcefully fight to get away. Sometimes I'll catch up and walk with her, other times I'll sit and talk to other people and wait for her as she returns from her rounds.

The only way to keep her in one place for any length of time seems to be to take her for rides. She still automatically fastens her own seat belt in the car, but cannot unfasten it.

In November, I attended a seminar that was being presented in Vista on the Y2K. One of the presenters, Loy Young, had recently moved to Vista. She had just finished writing a book entitled *The Plot–Victims, Villains and Heroes*, which I bought and read. Her explanation of the world made sense to me. I especially liked her insight about people and their behavior patterns. Of course, I had some questions about her theories, especially as it related to Sara's and my life. I e-mailed my questions to her, and resonated with her responses.

For the past couple of years I had been thinking of writing a book about Sara and her battle with Alzheimer's disease. But I never really pursued the idea because I wasn't a writer and had no knowledge of the publishing business. I asked Loy if she would look over the documentation that I had been keeping for some years and see if she would be interested in helping me with writing such a book.

After looking over my notes of the past few years, she said, "What you've written is a great foundation. You've carefully recorded the facts, which may in itself be of value to scientists that are doing research into Alzheimer's. To write a story though, I'll need to delve into your mind and know your thoughts about most of the events, as well as your feelings and reactions. You seem to be a very private man. Are you willing to go into the depths of your mind and your heart to find the answers to the questions I ask you? There could be pain on the way?" I wasn't so sure I fully understood what she was saying, but I already knew from reading her book that there was nothing superficial about her. If she could help me, I was willing to give it a try. She might have a point about my being too private. Sara, as well as the kids, often remarked that I kept too much to myself.

Prior to any formal negotiations, Loy wanted to visit Sara. I told her that Sara would not be able to talk to her. Loy just said, "There's much more to Sara than just her mind. I want to connect with her essence, her spirit and her feelings." One day I took her for a visit. It was a very quiet visit. I showed Loy around the nursing home, including Sara's room and introduced her to Linda, Sara's hairdresser. We sat out in front for a few minutes and Sara was able to name two trucks, which made us both happy.

Loy remarked, "Sara's easy to connect with. She's a gentle and caring soul. I believe she would indeed like for her story to be told. Beyond the ramifications of the disease or your role as a caregiver, there's a touching love story that's very inspiring. Would you be willing to tell me your love story?" I replied, "I don't see much about it that's inspiring, but I'll give it a try."

Monday, November 23, I received a message from the nursing home. Sara had been transported to a hospital emergency room. I went to the hospital to find Sara in the emergency room with an IV in her arm. Testing had shown that she was suffering from a urinary tract infection. The attending doctor said Sara would be in the hospital for at least a couple of days. After a couple of hours, Sara was moved from the emergency room into a regular hospital room. She seemed comfortable when I left.

Over the next couple of days Sara was still being medicated via an IV. She seemed comfortable. Corbin visited with me once.

On Wednesday night, November 25, I received a call from a nurse at the home saying, "Sara has been returned from the hospital. She is doing just fine and is walking around." For some reason I started crying. First time I had cried in quite awhile.

Thanksgiving morning I found Sara in her favorite corner of the dining room. We had our coffee and orange juice. She had no shoes, but instead was wearing hospital slippers. I checked with the nurse about the missing shoes and she said they would call the hospital and check to see where her shoes and clothes were. Sara went through a coughing spell, but otherwise seemed okay. Amy, Marc, Kyle and Ethan came home in the late afternoon. I prepared a Thanksgiving dinner for them.

We all went to visit Sara on Friday, after Thanksgiving. We found her asleep on a bed. She was shivering and had a red face. We took her to her own room and got a sweater for her. Her shoes were still missing.

On Saturday we visited again and found her asleep in her own bed. We sat and visited. Sara seemed unaware, as Kyle gave her some kisses. Still no shoes.

Sunday, Sara was in her favorite spot in the dining room. Still no shoes. The nurse had no information as to Sara's missing shoes. Sara was feeling better today. I got her to say, "Vern," and "Sara."

On Tuesday, I bought Sara some new shoes and took them to her. She was feeling much better, so we sat outside for awhile, then we walked around the nursing home.

Could not get her to name a truck or say a word.

Two weeks after being released from the hospital, I got a call from the nursing home telling me, "The hospital found Sara's shoes and clothing." I stopped by the hospital and picked up the shoes and clothes. I can't understand why it was so difficult to locate the clothing, it was in a bag with her name on it.

I presented Sara with a large birthday cake, enough to go around, for her sixty-third birthday. It made no impression on her, but the staff found it enjoyable. Birthdays, holidays and special occasions have no meaning for Sara anymore and haven't for some time.

> Sara is not feeling well, but she cannot tell anyone what is wrong. That's probably one of the worst things about the disease as it has progressed. Without being able to talk, she can't tell anyone the problems she's having. I'm sure many times her problems go on far too long before they are noticed. She's now fully assisted with most of the normal functions such as dressing, brushing her teeth, bowel movements and the like. She can still feed herself if the food is cut up and sometimes pull up the zipper on her jacket.
>
> Sara is tested for several things, including having a chest x-ray. She is looking sad and tired right now. Her constant slapping her thighs and clapping her hands annoys some of the other patients around her.

After nearly six weeks of negotiation on the book writing project, on December 23, Loy and I signed a four page contract for writing, *She Never Said Goodbye.* The book writing project would start the first week of January 1999, with a target date of completion of December 31, 1999.

On Christmas Day, Amy, Marc, Kyle, Ethan and I visited Sara. Corbin had to work and Darby was in Portland. During our visit, the duty nurse informed me, "Sara has been diagnosed as suffering from dehydration, which is one of the most common problems with Alzheimer's victims. Sara is now on an increased liquid intake, which is supposed to resolve the problem."

It was just a quiet Christmas Day at home. As it should be, Kyle was the one seeming to enjoy it the most.

On December 27, my 64th birthday, I had bronchitis so bad I could not visit Sara. Amy and crew went down and reported that Sara pushed Ethan around in his stroller. Amy said she had taken some orange juice and that Sara drank it all. They apparently had a very nice visit.

I received a call from the nursing home on the morning of December 30, saying, "Sara has a cracked tooth and needs to see a dentist." I called our dentist and made arrangements to get Sara in on an emergency basis. It took me ten minutes to find Sara when I arrived at the nursing home. We went to the dentist, where we had to wait for forty-five minutes. Sara kept hitting herself quite hard. She would not cooperate with the dentist, which was unusual, and made things rather difficult.

It turned out she did not have a cracked tooth at all, just some food stuck in her teeth. I reported this fact back to the nurses who had no explanation other then what they thought they had observed.

I got home at around 3:30 p.m. At about 5:00 p.m. I got a call from the nursing home indicating that Sara was on her way, by ambulance, to Palomar Hospital emergency room in Escondido. This was rather upsetting news! Of course I had questions, such as "Why was she being sent to an emergency room?" I had just left her a short time before and she was fine. "Why all the way to Palomar Hospital in Escondido, rather than across the street to Scripps in Encinitas? Who ordered this action?"

The nurse said, "Dr. Newhous ordered Sara taken to the ER and you need to talk to him." So I called Dr. Newhous, who said, "The nurses wanted Sara examined." He said, "I told the nurse I would not be able to see Sara until after the first of the year and the nurses wanted her examined before then." I told him, "She's gone through all kinds of tests earlier in the month, of which you are aware. On Christmas Day I was told she was suffering from dehydration and remedial action was being taken." Dr. Newhous just said again, that the nurses wanted her seen by a doctor and he wasn't available.

Shortly after talking to Dr. Newhous, I got a call from the ambulance, enroute to Palomar Hospital, the ambulance person told me, "We've been informed that the Palomar ER is too busy and we are now heading for Pomerado Hospital ER in Poway." I was becoming incensed! Here it was a Wednesday night during rush hour and Sara being driven all over North County San Diego. For what reason?

I called Dr. Newhous and told him what was going on with the ambulance and gave him the phone number of the ambulance enroute to Poway.

Dr. Newhous called back and told me, "The ambulance has just gotten to the Pomerado Hospital ER and I've talked to a doctor there. Sara will be going back to the nursing home shortly."

At 9:15 p.m., Sara was released from the emergency room and was returned to the nursing home.

It took several weeks to find out what all happened on this night. Without a power of attorney, I would not have been allowed to get the information I needed.

Dr. Newhous said, "It was the nurses who wanted her sent to the ER." The nurses said, "It was Dr. Newhous who wanted her sent to the ER." The report of the visit to the ER, at a cost of $900, showed that tests conducted there were basically identical to those conducted earlier in the month. The ER report indicated that Dr. Newhous was supposed to follow up on the case in five days, which he did not.

The ER visit resulted in absolutely nothing in the way of treatment of Sara for anything. The nursing home did not receive any information from the hospital ER until early February 1999. Dr. Newhous' office never produced any results from the ER visit.

I had a discussion with the director of the nursing home in which he basically stated, "We have no control over what a doctor orders." He also told me that obtaining results of ER visits is not their responsibility, but that of the doctor ordering a patient to the ER. Whether it was the doctor or the nursing home's screw up, I may never know.

After nearly four years in the nursing home, this had to be the most upsetting thing to happen concerning Sara's care. I guess it's a good thing that Sara did not understand what was going on as she rode around in the ambulance that night. What a way to end the year!

Chapter 24

My Love is Eternal

y visit to Sara on New Year's Day 1999 found her lying on a bed. I coaxed and asked, "Please get up and visit with me." No response. I finally helped her by gently taking her hands and pulling her up and off the bed. I gave her orange juice and we sat inside. Today Sara could not say one word, even with my prodding.

The first week in January 1999, I began writing *She Never Said Goodbye*. My first step was to sort through all of our letters and put them in chronological order. Sara and I are both sentimental and have kept most of the letters that we wrote each other during our courtship, as well as our marriage when I was away in Vietnam and Okinawa.

Sara's mother also kept all of Sara's correspondence through the years, as did Amy, our youngest daughter, who kept letters her mother wrote to her while she was in college. We had recorded over ten thousand feet of home movies as the children were growing up.

It looks as if I will be walking down a path of nostalgia for some months to come.

Every morning, Monday through Friday, I worked on the book with my co-author, I must admit sometimes I got really frustrated. Writing about an event wasn't enough for Loy, she wanted to know what I thought about it, what I felt about it, and if I had any physical reactions. Feelings were the most difficult for me to come up with, so she made up a list for me. After a while, it became apparent that Loy was going to know more about me than anyone in my life had, maybe even myself.

I visited Sara on Tuesday and Thursday afternoons and Saturday and Sunday mornings. I noticed that I was becoming more aware of Sara's feelings, as I became aware of mine.

On January 29, I flew to Colorado for a surprise 70th birthday party for a friend of mine of many years, Ray Stephens. On my first visit with Sara, after my return, she seemed quite happy . . . even with her diapers down to her knees. After getting the diapers back in place, we sat out front. I am no longer bothered by Sara's urinary or fecal incontinence.

Today I got her to say "Vern," which seemed to make her happy momentarily. Whenever she is able to say even one word like my name or naming a truck, it does seem to give her a brief second of pleasure. Then it's back to her usual silence.

Our days are pretty much routine. My visits usually start the same, trying to find Sara. If she isn't walking the halls, I check her favorite spot in the recreation room. If she isn't there, then I check the beds in every room, until I find her. Sometimes she's asleep, other times just lying on the bed. Of course if I arrive at mealtime, it's not a problem finding her.

We spend most of our time together sitting out front of the nursing home on a bench where we can see the freeway. Some days she can name a truck, other days none. As time passes, she rarely ever names a truck. In fact, she will go days upon days without even being able to speak one word, requiring me to find other ways to relate with Sara. Its like a presenter at a seminar Loy and I attended, who said something to the effect that Alzheimer's victims, in the late stages, are like a person in a house with the light on— you know they are there, as the light is on— but when you ring the bell, they can't come to the door—that doesn't mean they aren't home!

I continue to bring Sara orange juice unless I arrive at mealtime. I have no expectation of whether she will drink it or not. Some days she will hardly touch it and others she will take it and drink it quickly. In the end, I guess what matters is that I enjoy bringing the orange juice to her. All throughout our marriage, I've delighted in bringing her gifts, small and large. Now, about the only thing I really can bring her, besides clothes, is the orange juice, and occasionally a burger or a milkshake.

Sara is becoming more and more consistent with the hand clapping, slapping her legs and rocking back and forth. Some days will be more dramatic than others. Occasionally there are quiet days, but they are rare.

On March 21, Darby, her husband, Brad, and his two daughters, arrived from Oregon for a week's visit. It was to be a week of playing tourist. One day Darby, Brad, Corbin and I visited Sara together. I tried to help Sara say their names, but she was unable to formulate words. When I asked her where Corbin was, she didn't respond verbally. She communicated non verbally, with her body, by turning and looking at him with recognition.

Late March, the nursing home started another remodeling project. This time it was to divide the main dining room, which also served as a recreation room, into two separate rooms. One room would be used strictly for dining and the other as a recreation room to be used for both activities and dining. The remodeling project would cause Sara to lose her favorite spot at which to sit. She soon adopted a new favorite location in the new recreation room where her favorite sofa had been relocated.

Due to Sara's clapping and slapping, which disturbed other patients, she and a select small group of others ate their meals in a small separate room near the nurse's station.

It wasn't possible to segregate Sara at all times though, and her clapping and slapping had become a real annoyance to some of the other patients. In fact, on March 26, I got a call from the nursing home, the nurse said, "I need to report that one of the female patients slapped Sara on her rear, three or four times." Luckily Sara was not injured. The hitting was apparently in retaliation for Sara's hand clapping.

The book writing is coming along slowly but surely. Amazingly, I wrote over 140,000 words of memoirs of Sara's and my life, spanning six decades. *She Never Said Goodbye* is only a few chapters of our memoirs.

My mood changed as I began to revisit happier times in our life. My sadness often lifted for the few hours that we wrote, sometimes spilling over into the day.

Other days, as I revisited some really hurtful times, my sadness was almost overwhelming. I don't know if I would have continued if I had been doing it by myself. Maybe that's why I never wrote the book myself, to begin with. I hadn't realized how deeply depressed I was. One day I wept for myself as I realized that as Sara had begun to die, so had I.

Shortly thereafter, I started gardening again, which I found helpful. I've gardened, when I've had the chance, throughout my life, but when Sara got so bad, I quit. I've always enjoyed watching vegetables and flowers emerging out of the ground with new life.

May 13, I got another call from the nursing home saying, "Sara has been hit by another patient as a result of her hand clapping. She's not hurt, maybe stunned, if anything." Poor Sara, I knew the nursing home couldn't watch all of the patients every moment. Certainly I understood how her constant clapping and slapping could indeed be disturbing to other patients, it was often disturbing to me just for the time I was with her.

All I could do was to take Sara to see Dr. Smith for further evaluation of her medication. The medication was supposed to help control her agitation and clapping and slapping. The results were not apparent. He increased her Resperidone from .5mg to 1.0mg, morning and evening.

Sara was doing a good job of feeding herself now. You would have never known that at one time she couldn't feed herself. Her ability to handle a fork and spoon was good, although she did need help cutting her food.

Over the years, Sara has taken just about every drug associated with controlling the impulses of Alzheimer's victims. On our next visit to Dr. Smith, he changed Sara's medication from Resperidone to Clonedine.

On June 17, my co-writer, Loy, and her mother, Violet, went with me to see Sara. A member of their family, Loy's aunt and Violet's sister in law has late onset Alzheimer's and is in a home in Oklahoma. More and more I hear of people, like myself, with a member of their family suffering from Alzheimer's. Just think, a short time ago, I knew nothing about it. Now it's being heralded as the disease of the coming century.

First we visited Sara's room and then went and sat on the patio. Sara communicated by looking at both of them and smiling. She even said "Vern," which was the first word she had said in weeks. For just a moment Sara smiled and acted really pleased with herself. Certainly brightened up my day!

Sara also wet her pants that day, which happened often, so we took her to the nurse for a change. Sara didn't appear to be bothered about wetting her pants, and neither did I anymore.

Amy and Ethan came down on June 19 for a two day visit. We visited Sara at which time she got to hold Ethan. When Sara clapped her hands, Ethan joined right in by mimicking her and clapping his. He thought that was great fun. Even with my prodding, Sara wasn't able to say any names that day, however, when I asked her if she liked her orange juice, she was able to say, "Yes."

I've read that yes or no will probably be the last words she will utter. Even though it drove me crazy at the time, I do miss the, "I love you," and, "You're special."

One day a new development occurred. Sara began slapping her chest. It was the first time I had witnessed this action. She still claps her hands and slaps her legs but it varies from day to day as to the intensity and frequency.

On July 9, I picked up Sara to take her to see Dr. Smith for a medication check. When I arrived at the nursing home it was apparent that someone had just died. There was a hospice person there, and the staff was cleaning personal property out of a room. When Sara and I returned from seeing Dr. Smith, there was a man in the hallway crying and being consoled by staff. I never determined who died.

I had difficulty finding her on one visit. Then suddenly I heard her clapping, and I knew that was my Sara. The clapping led me straight to her. She was lying on a bed just clapping away, with her eternal smile on her face. I was glad to find her.

One day at lunch, I was talking to one of the nursing assistants. She reported that the Alzheimer's unit was short six nursing assistants, thus she was working a double shift. There are six nursing assistants on every shift, as well as two nurses. Over the years I have seen many prospective employees filling out employment applications in the area of the reception desk. The nursing assistant informed me, "The starting pay is $8.20 an hour and could be higher, depending upon experience. Some prospective employees get eliminated when they fail background checks." It seems a prior drug history eliminates anyone.

Sometime later I heard on the radio that in the year 2000 there could be a shortage of 30,000 nurses or certified nursing assistants in California. The shortage is a result, supposedly, of low Medi-Cal payments, by the state, to nursing homes. If sufficient new employees cannot be hired, it could become a crisis, nursing homes may have to reject admitting new patients.

Things at the nursing home have changed a great deal in the nearly five years that Sara has been there. Probably the most significant change has been the condition of the patients being admitted. When Sara was admitted in February of 1995, it was a requirement that she be able to walk. As the director of the nursing home, Mrs. Watkins, pointed out to me one day, now they are admitting patients in wheelchairs. One day in the new recreation room I took a count and found only nine patients who could walk, unassisted. Twenty-two others were in wheelchairs or what they called "merrywalkers."

One of the nursing assistants informed me, "The wheelchairs and merrywalkers are fine for those using them, but are a hazard to the patients who can still walk, they find it difficult to dodge around the wheelchairs and merrywalkers which could lead to falls." At least for now, Sara is able to walk quite well.

I took a mental note one day on who was "missing." In my mind I noted several patients who I had not seen over several days or weeks. I knew two of them had died and would assume the others did too, if they had not been transferred to the skilled nursing wing due to injury or illness.

In late August, Amy, and family, came down for a visit. Neither Kyle nor Ethan would let Sara hold them. I'm always hoping when the family is there that Sara can recognize them or say a word. Today, even with all the coaxing that I did, she was not able to say a word.

The following day, Sara and I were sitting out front, having our coffee and orange juice, when she said, "Ryder," as one of their trucks passed! It was the first word she had said in over two months. Amazing how the recognition of a truck and a word can uplift Sara's spirits for a moment—but mine all day long.

My last visit, as I end this chapter, was to visit Sara with my co-writer and an associate of hers, Francine Dufour, who made a video of us.

I had Linda Dixon, the hairdresser, fix Sara's hair. At sixty-three, Sara amazingly has almost no gray hair which makes her age seem much younger. Linda put lipstick on Sara and even did her nails. I must say Sara still looks beautiful. If you saw her from afar, you wouldn't even know anything was wrong.

We threw the giant plastic ball back and forth to each other for almost ten minutes before she lost interest. I wonder if somewhere in her mind she's still playing tennis and the ball has just gotten bigger.

Then we went to Sara's room where we played some music Sara had taped, that was popular during our years of growing up, such as *Accentuate the Positive, Don't Get Around Much Anymore* and *Don't Sit Under the Apple Tree.* We danced for a few moments before she lay down on her bed clapping to the music. Sara was still able to follow my lead, ever so slowly.

We took this music to her since we had recently learned at an Alzheimer's conference that even patients like Sara, who no longer have the ability to recognize their loved ones, have reached incontinence, and are unable to speak, can still respond with other senses. They can respond to music, especially if it's of their childhood and young adult years. Also they respond to aroma therapy and to art.

During the year I've been writing this book, new scientific discoveries are being made all the time. To me, the most profound discovery has been that the brain cells can indeed regenerate. One day when someone like Sara is diagnosed with Alzheimer's, hopefully the doctor won't have to say, "The brain is in a state of deterioration and nothing can be done."

The second most exciting discovery I've heard of this past year is that a bacterium has been found in the autopsies of the brains of Alzheimer's patients. The bacterium causes respiratory infections such as pneumonia. They've already found a vaccine that showed good results in mice, undoubtedly they will start research on humans soon. The idea of a bacterium causing respiratory infections in Alzheimer's patients made sense to me, as one of my biggest questions has been, "What do Alzheimer's patients die of?"

While interviewing Sara's mother, Grammy, about the book, she told Loy, "Sara almost died when she was one year old from pneumonia." I know that all through our marriage Sara was susceptible to upper respiratory infections and continues to be treated, now and then, for upper respiratory infections in the nursing home.

As one way of coping with Sara's condition, our youngest daughter, Amy, has learned to daydream. Her favorite daydream is of Sara walking out of the nursing home, after ten years, and being awarded a million dollars for her contribution to the advancement of a cure for Alzheimer's. Haven't we all been taught to dream the impossible dream and to believe in miracles?

I've learned to dream myself, to keep our love alive. I also dream about resolving the nagging thought in my mind of our home going to the state when I die. Maybe, through the proceeds from this book, I can reimburse the state for Sara's nursing home expenses. I'll give it my best, then I'll be satisfied.

****

Right now though, in the present, I'm ensuring that I notice, and appreciate, the small things. I'm enjoying watching her walk, as one day she will no longer be able to walk, but will be in a "merrywalker" herself, instead of just dodging them. Today I'm appreciating that she can sit upright in a chair. One day I may find that she can no longer sit upright, but will have to lie down. Today I'm grateful that she can hold her head up and look at me. One of the final losses is the inability to hold up ones head.

Luckily what I love most, the smile, is the last to go. Even when her smile goes, I hope to be able to connect with the smile of her spirit as she disengages from her body. My love for Sara is not just for now, it's eternal.

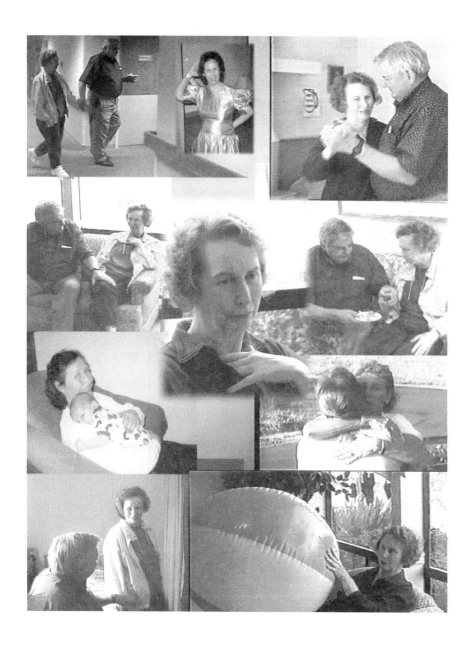

Ten Ways to Keep Your Love Alive

- Return smiles and hugs

- Sign both of your names when you write to family and friends

- Continue giving appropriate gifts because you like to give, not because you are expecting them to be appreciated

- Keep a picture of your loved one in happier times by your bed or at your desk so you see it daily

- Include your loved one in conversations with friends and family

- Sit quietly together and enjoy your loved one's presence

- Share family pictures with your loved one, even if they may not show outward signs of recognition

- Continue to celebrate your special days, like birthdays and wedding anniversaries

- Believe there will be a cure in their lifetime

- Dream

Helpful Information

This helpful information section offers factors that readers might wish to consider in planning their lives.

Unfortunately in our case, we had no warning and had never thought of the subject of long-term illness and long-term care. The Alzheimer's Association has compelling evidence indicating the disease may be present as long as 20 to 40 years before the first clinical symptoms appear.

This summary might be taken as a warning, to consider what can, and will, happen to millions in the not too distant future.

Is It Alzheimer's?

Alzheimer's is a form of dementia, but dementia can take many forms and have different causes. It is true that Alzheimer's disease is the most common form of dementia in the elderly. However, the definition of "elderly" can vary significantly and often is in the eyes of the observer. I certainly did not consider Sara elderly in her fifties.

In Sara's case, my initial thought was that she had a case of depression. That was the initial diagnosis for which treatment was commenced. No thought whatsoever was given to Alzheimer's. But eventually as no improvement was noted and in fact deterioration continued, further evaluation commenced. Psychiatric and psychological examinations were conducted. Various neurological and laboratory tests were also conducted. This took months and no medical authority would actually say the dreaded word "Alzheimer's." But in the end, by a process of elimination and the medications prescribed, even I could deduce that Sara suffered from Alzheimer's. Although Alzheimer's can only be confirmed by autopsy after death, the medical profession has gotten to the stage they can quite accurately diagnose Alzheimer's in 80 to 90 percent of the cases. It's getting them to diagnose it early-on that is the problem. I'm hopeful that the information contained herein proves helpful to others in considering Alzheimer's as the reason for the disturbing behaviors in those less than elderly.

Memory loss, confusion, impaired judgment, or changes in behavior for no apparent reason should sound a warning bell to those around a person displaying these symptoms of dementia. Early medical evaluation is important for all concerned. The diagnosis of some kind of dementia, especially Alzheimer's, can create the need to make many decisions regarding medical care, finances, legal matters, and personal planning. One of the first decisions I recommend is to contact a local chapter of the Alzheimer's Association for advice and assistance.

Following are a few of the effective programs and strategies that helped me in the role of caregiver:

"Safe Return"

Safe Return is a national program started in 1993. It assists in identifying and returning to their caregivers those persons suffering from dementia who wander away. Caregivers are human and on occasion the dementia victim may escape from their care and become lost. The Safe Return program is certainly recommended for persons identified with dementia who are ambulatory.

Safe Return has grown significantly and has become more sophisticated over the years. Law enforcement agencies are being brought into the program through training provided by the Alzheimer's Association. There were over 53,000 enrollees as of 1999. Sara was one of the first enrollees and even though she is now in a locked facility, I maintain her enrollment and she still wears her Safe Return bracelet.

The Alzheimer's Association does not know how many dementia victims have wandered away only to be found dead days, weeks, or months later. I know here in San Diego County I have read of three such cases.

LEARNING SEMINARS

For years when opening the morning paper, I would find flyers announcing free seminars on various subjects involving financial planning. Topics included Medicaid, Medi-Cal (California), Medicare, long-term care insurance, avoiding probate, conservatorship, death taxes, preservation of family assets, long-term nursing home costs, avoiding capital gains taxes, dangers of joint tenancy, living trusts, increasing your present income, paying less taxes and reducing risks to present investments. Attorneys, financial planners, and insurance representatives generally host these workshops. You can learn a great deal at these presentations, particularly if you have no previous knowledge of these subjects. Always keep in mind that these workshops may be free until such time you decide to buy or invest in one of the many products usually made available. As part of anyone's normal financial planning, I would certainly encourage everyone to take advantage of these seminars, particularly if your knowledge is limited on financial subjects. Just consider it continuing education.

Laws are continually changing in these categories and in some instances will vary from state to state, but it is a place to start, and the seminars are usually free. As a little bonus, they even have free coffee and pastries at most presentations.

ALZHEIMER'S ASSOCIATION

In Sara's case, I did not have the information I would have liked to have at the time her life started to break down. The initial diagnosis of pre-senile dementia avoided the more descriptive term Alzheimer's disease. Thus I stumbled along with her care and my planning for over a year without professional assistance. I did not become aware of the Alzheimer's Association until her case had progressed significantly. I was never advised by anyone, [including her doctors,] to contact this helpful association for assistance and advice.

The Alzheimer's Association is a relatively new national organization when compared to the national heart, cancer, and diabetes associations. Originally founded in 1980, the Alzheimer's

Association has grown significantly over the past 20 years. It has over 200 local chapters. There are also over 1,600 support groups nationwide and like all charitable organizations, they must compete for donations.

The local chapters provide extensive information to those who request it. They can provide a list of lawyers specializing in elder law, along with a list of legal issues that caregivers should consider. They do not recommend specific lawyers, but at least they provide a starting point. They can also provide a list of medical personnel who are familiar with the diagnosis and treatment of Alzheimer's disease, but again, they make no endorsements.

At least once a year the San Diego Association provides a seminar on the legal concerns of caregivers. It was not until I contributed to the Alzheimer's Association and was entered on their mailing list that I learned about things I would have liked to have known much earlier.

Support Groups

There are many support groups for Alzheimer's caregivers. Your local Alzheimer's Association can provide a list of dates, times, and locations of support group meetings. This could be a good place to seek referrals for legal, medical, and financial personnel.

Long-Term Care

The term "care" can take on different meanings. An article by Michael Prince in the January 29, 1998, issue of Business Insurance entitled "Elder Care Benefits Valued: Demand for Benefits Expected to Grow" predicts that elder care will replace child care as the number one dependent care issue in the United States by 2005. One out of three workers will be caring for an aging family member. In most instances this would be defined as long-term care.

Most people think long-term care involves only the elderly. However, according to the American Academy of Actuaries Long-Term Care: Actuarial Issues in Designing Voluntary Federal-Private LTC Programs, January 1999, 40 percent of those receiving long-term care are working age adults between 18 and 64 years of age.

Automobile accidents, work related injuries, sports injuries, and various diseases lead to an overlooked need for long-term care among many younger Americans.

Will long-term care be there when you need it? For the rich, the cost of long-term care may not be a concern. Kiplinger's Personal Finance Magazine, May 1997, indicates that the average cost of nursing home care is more than $46,000 a year. The cost of a stay in a nursing home can vary significantly with location. The Wall Street Journal, March 31, 1999, notes that costs can range from $40,000 to $100,000 a year. It is easy to see that the assets of a middle class family would not last long bearing that kind of expense. I know, I have been there.

Long-term care is more often provided at home, but it can still be costly. For the poor, long-term care may not be a financial problem as long as Medicaid remains viable. Long-term care costs really must be considered carefully by the middle class, the definition of which varies according to one's income and assets. Middle class in the eyes of one observer or politician may vary with the next observer or politician.

I consider the middle class to be a group that has managed to work hard and accumulate some assets that will carry them comfortably through their retirement years. They may have planned well and saved wisely for their golden years. They may have a good private health plan or a good Medicare supplement. It is this middle class group that must look long and carefully at the need for long-term care insurance. But again one must ask, when do they look? At what age do long-term care concerns come into focus?

It is easy to see that it's impractical to apply for fire insurance for your home after it has burned to the ground. Trying to get automobile insurance after your car has been totaled in an accident is not an option. Long-term care insurance is not available to those who have been identified as needing it.

Insurance for any purpose may never be needed. But people buy insurance because it may be needed. As a part of good financial planning families often pay for life, health, accident, automobile, and homeowner's insurance. The young seldom take out long-term care insurance. Long-term care insurance is something for "old" people and when you are young, old is a long way away.

Long-term care insurance can be expensive, particularly if provided for both spouses and possibly other family members. One should remember that long-term care requirements could be the result of factors other than just old age, and other family members may benefit from long-term care insurance, as well.

As I mentioned in the text of the book, after assisting me in admitting Sara to the nursing home and seeing what I would be going through financially, my brother and his wife immediately applied for and were accepted for long-term care insurance. They saw a need.

I also applied for and was accepted for long-term care insurance. There are all kinds of long-term care insurance plans. I picked one that I thought suited my needs.

Loy Young, the co-author of this book, who is still in her fifties, has learned a great deal by her participation in this writing effort. Not long after the writing project commenced, she realized the value of long-term care insurance, and applied. She had a concussion a couple of years ago and had a very difficult time before being accepted.

We learned from her insurance agent, Mr. Paul Riddle, a licensed attorney and insurance broker in California and a specialist in long-term care insurance, that approximately 10 percent of all applications for long-term health care insurance are denied. Coverage may be denied for what sometimes seem like ridiculous reasons, but the fact is when you are denied you must make alternative plans.

Mr. Riddle indicated that the median age for receiving benefits from long-term care insurance is eighty-two years of age. The most common reason people are rejected is that they waited too long and didn't apply until they already required assistance in their daily living. He does his own initial screening of applicants. He noted that if you have oxygen available in your home you most probably would be turned down. If you are already in a wheelchair, you may be accepted, but only at the highest possible rate. Other reasons for rejection are head injuries or a combination of problems like high blood pressure, diabetes, and numbness in the limbs. Like nursing homes, insurance companies don't have to approve your application. It's a business.

People buy long-term care insurance, Mr. Riddle says, for a few reasons. First, many people do not want to turn family members into nurses who must feed, bathe, and clothe them. People also want to prevent the loss of their assets. Another common reason appears to be the ability to choose where they will go, because the long-term care insurance makes a nicer place more affordable.

Any thought given to the use of Medicaid for long-term care must be evaluated closely. Although the nursing home in which Sara resides accepts Medicaid (Medi-Cal), at last report there was a two year waiting list.

Mr. Riddle noted that financial planners are legally required to suggest long-term care insurance to their clients in California. Many people will need long-term care well before their elder years. It's a big gamble. When young, most people believe they will live forever. When old, most die before their time.

Long-term care insurance is not for everybody, but is it for you? The October 1997 issue of *Consumer Reports* has an excellent article on long-term care insurance.

THE PENDING HEALTH CARE CRISIS

Starting in November 1999, the California Association of Health Facilities sponsored a public announcement via radio of a pending nursing home crisis in California. The crisis is the result of a lack of Certified Nursing Assistants (CNA's) to meet the growing needs of the nursing home industry. In early 2000, California could face a shortage of 30,000 CNA's. The shortage is the result of the low pay earned by CNA's who work in a very demanding and stressful environment. If new CNA's cannot be recruited in the numbers needed, the result could be that growing numbers of those needing nursing home care will be turned away.

Alzheimer's is being called "The Disease of the Century," its impact on the nursing home industry threatens to be of colossal proportions.

LAWYERS

One time I heard that the average American would have to seek legal advice (i.e., see a lawyer) eleven times in his or her life. That was many years ago and at the time I had never had the need to see a lawyer. I thought it was rather bizarre to think of needing to see a lawyer eleven times on the average in a lifetime. Subsequently I have exceeded the average of eleven times in a rather short period of time.

Lawyers come in all shapes, races, sexes, knowledge, interests, and most importantly, competence. Lawyers most often advance their expertise in certain parts of the law: business law, divorce law, real estate law, etc., and some specialize in elder law, medical law, long-term care law, etc. The Alzheimer's Association can provide you with a list of lawyers who specialize in elder law and Medicaid eligibility.

But how do you know if the lawyer you feel you need at the time is the right one for you? Of course the number one way is to get a referral. A referral may come from a friend or a relative, but I would strongly suggest it be from someone who has gone through what you are about to go through and was satisfied with the legal assistance they received.

What services would you want from a lawyer? Everyone's needs are different. Things to consider might include a durable power of attorney, a living trust, wills, and a durable power of attorney for health care, a quit claim deed, a community property agreement and an agreement to sever joint tenancies. Advice regarding long-term care insurance (if it is not too late) and qualifying for Medicaid are other considerations.

MEDICAID

What is Medicaid? Title XIX of the Social Security Act is a program that provides medical assistance for certain individuals and families with low income and financial resources. The Medicaid program became law in 1965 as a jointly funded cooperative venture between the federal and state governments to assist states in the provision of adequate medical care to eligible needy persons. Medicaid is the largest national program providing medical and health related services to the poorest people. Within broad national guidelines provided by the federal government, each of the states establishes its own eligibility standards, determines the type, amount, duration, and scope of services, sets the rate of payment for services, and administers its own program.

In California, Medicaid is known as Medi-Cal. As noted, although similar in most respects, each state's Medicaid program may vary slightly from the other states.

In 1995, 4.4 million elderly were beneficiaries of Medicaid. It is estimated that two-thirds of all elderly in nursing homes are Medicaid beneficiaries. However, it is also estimated that 85 percent of those receiving long-term care are not in nursing homes and may not be elderly. According to the Journal of Financial Planning, March 1999, it is estimated that 43 percent of Americans over age 65 will spend some time in a nursing home during their lifetime.

Many members of middle class families have qualified for Medicaid only after spending down their assets for long-term care, either in their own home or in a nursing home. The Balanced Budget Act of 1997 (BBA) authorized the Program of All-Inclusive Care for the Elderly (PACE) which features a comprehensive service delivery system and integrated Medicare and Medicaid financing. This program is designed to provide long-term care at home rather than in an institution.

MEDICAID EXPERTS

There are also other professionals who help individuals learn about and deal with Medicaid. I was fortunate to obtain the services of an expert in Medi-Cal, California's version of Medicaid. He was an expert on all issues related to Medi-Cal procedures and qualifications, although not a lawyer. He had been a social services worker handling Medi-Cal cases for the state.

The paperwork needed to gain Sara's eligibility amounted to over 130 pages and having an expert to work with made the final submission significantly easier.

POWER OF ATTORNEY

One of the most important documents a caregiver should have is a durable power of attorney over the everyday affairs of the Alzheimer's victim. Such a document must be finalized while the Alzheimer's victim is still capable and legally able to provide it. An easy solution is just to complete this document between man and wife while both are still well. The question sometimes arises, how much do you trust your spouse or relative? It is a powerful document.

DURABLE POWER OF ATTORNEY FOR HEALTH CARE

I suggest people look carefully at their own outlooks and beliefs pertaining to health care in catastrophic circumstances. A durable power of attorney for health care gives control of health decisions to a pre authorized person when one becomes unable to make them for oneself. It is a powerful document that allows people to specify the type of care they would or would not like to have performed on their behalf.

WEBSITES

Over the past few years, the number and scope of Internet Websites that provide important information on health related issues have expanded greatly. A few Web sites that may be of interest to the reader are listed below:

ALZHEIMER'S ASSOCIATION

This is a good starting place for those needing information on Alzheimer's. The site offers tips on caregiving, updates on research and treatments, and information on programs and services provided by local chapters. 1.800.272.3900.

http://www.alz.org

ALZHEIMER'S DISEASE EDUCATION AND REFERRAL CENTER (ADEAR)

Center for Research and clinical trials. 1.800.438.4380.

http://www.alzheimers.org

FAMILY CAREGIVER ALLIANCE

Practical information on care giving and related matters. 1.415.434.3388.

http://www.caregiver.org

CAREGIVER NETWORK (CANADA)

Information on home care, housing, medical issues, care giving, and dementia in Canada.

http://www.caregiver.on.ca

HEALTH CARE FINANCING ADMINISTRATION (HCFA)

The federal agency that administers the Medicare, Medicaid, and Child Health Insurance programs. Provides extensive information on these services. 1.410.786.3000.

http://www.hcfa.gov

NATIONAL INSTITUTES OF HEALTH (NIH)

The mission of NIH is to uncover new knowledge that will lead to better health for everyone.

http://www.nih.gov

NATIONAL INSTITUTE ON AGING (NIA)

Part of the National Institutes of Health, the NIA is the principal biomedical research agency of the U.S. Government. It promotes healthy aging by conducting and supporting biomedical, social, and behavioral research and public education. 1.301.496.1752.

http://www.nih.gov/nia

MEDICAID PROGRAM

Provides in depth information on the Medicaid program.
http://www.hcfa.gov/medicaid/mover.htm

CAREGIVER WEB SITE

Useful information for caregivers.
http://www.webofcare.com

THE GEORGE G. GLENNER ALZHEIMER'S FAMILY CENTERS, INC.

The George G. Glenner Alzheimer's Family Centers, Inc. School of Dementia Care and four Adult Day Care Centers (San Diego, Escondido, Chula Vista, Fallbrook). Affiliated with the University of California, San Diego School of Medicine, Alzheimer's Research Center. Free Alzheimer's video and booklet in English and Spanish, "Living in Alzheimer's Disease." Telephone 1.800.736.6674.

RECOMMENDED READING

The 36-Hour Day, by Nancy L. Mace, M.A. and Peter V. Rabins, M.D., M.P.H., 1981, 1991 by the Johns Hopkins University Press.

Index

The Author

George Vernon Ellison is the beloved husband of Sara. They have been married for thirty-seven years. His life has been one of service. Vern retired as a Major with twenty years in the Marine Corps, and spent seventeen years in the California Community College system teaching and coaching at Palomar College in San Marcos. He continues to take care of Sara and is still a devoted father and grandfather. Vern envisions his future as one in which he is influential in educating the public and helping people become aware of Alzheimer's and the effect it can have on a family.

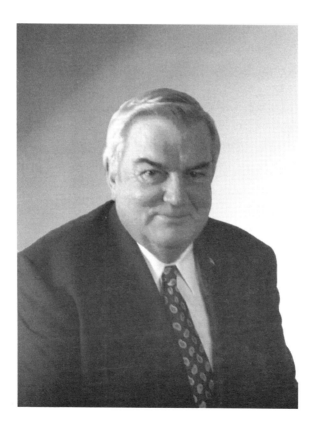

The Co-Author

L oy Young participated in this book as a co-author and writer's coach. She has authored twenty-two other books. Her book, *The Plot—Victims, Villains and Heroes*, is a must read for those understanding the vast world of feelings and global human behavior. For more information visit websites: www.RelationshipTrainingCenter.com and www.AquariusHousePress.com

DEDICATION:

Although this story is about Sara and Vern Ellison, its reminiscent of stories about my beloved Aunt Reath who suffers from Alzheimer's and is in a nursing home in Oklahoma. It's also about her husband of over fifty years, my Uncle Buck and his struggle as a caregiver. I dedicate my work on this book to both of them and also to those throughout the world who struggle with this ravaging disease as well as to all of their caregivers.

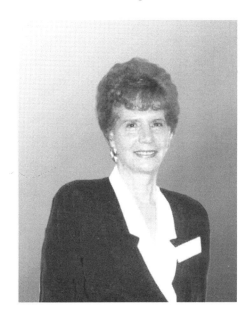

Artist

Francine Dufour participated in this book as the photographer, cover designer, illustrator, and artist. Francine has been an artist her entire life. Although her repertoire includes original oil painting and reproductions, her latest passion is silk painting. Her work can be viewed on-line at www.RelationshipTrainingCenter.com and in Vista, CA, at Vision Art Gallery.

Francine's intent, as a person and as an artist, is to see, appreciate, and then express, the beauty and spirit in the world and the cosmos.

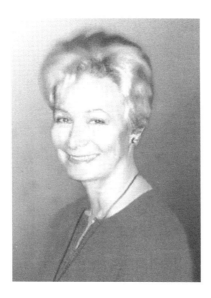

If you would like to buy additional copies of *She Never Said Goodbye* by mail, please fill out this order form and send it along with a check or money order, payable to:

Aquarius House Press
PO Box 1241
Vista, California 92085

If you would like to purchase by credit card go to the website: www.AquariusHousePress.com to order on-line, or phone Aquarius House Press at 760.758.7004. Questions? Email to sales@AquariusHousePress.com—orders by E-mail: send credit card number, expiration date, name on the card along with number of copies wanted.

PRICES
Hardback $24.95 + (California Residents) Sales Tax $1.93
Paperback $19.95 + (California Residents) Sales Tax $1.55

S & H $3.50 for one book
$1.50 for each additional book at same address.

There is a ten per cent discount for orders of ten or more.

Vern Ellison is using his profits from the book to reimburse the state for Sara's nursing home care which will secure his home to the family trust for his children and grandchildren.

Send this book to:
Name_____
Address_____
City_____Sate_____ Zip_____

Send another book to:
Name_____
Address_____
City_____Sate_____ Zip_____